Change
of Life

Change of Life

The Menopause Handbook

by

Susan Flamholtz Trien

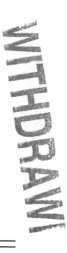

Fawcett Columbine • New York

To David, Stacey and Adam,
my live-in support group.

A Fawcett Columbine Book
Published by Ballantine Books

Copyright © 1986 by Susan Flamholtz Trien
Illustrations copyright © 1986 by Elaine Yabroudy

The author is grateful for permission to quote from the following previously
published material:

Ellen Goodman. "Gary Makes Her Feel Young Again." Copyright © 1984,
The Boston Globe Newspaper Company/Washington Post Writers Group,
reprinted with permission.

E. Kathryn McGoldrick. "Myths, Menopause and Middle Age." *Journal of
the American Medical Women's Association*, Vol. 37, No. 4 (April 1982),
p. 86.

Diane Alington-Mackinnon and Lillian E. Troll. "The Adaptive Function
of the Menopause: A Devil's Advocate Position." *The Journal of the American Geriatric Society*, Vol. 29, No. 8 (August 1981), pp. 349-353.

Gail Sheehy. *Pathfinders*. William Morrow & Co., New York, 1981.

Ann M. Voda. "Hot Flushes/Flashes . . . A Descriptive Analysis." *Menopause Update*, Vol. 1, No. 2 (1983), p. 17.

Library of Congress Catalog Card Number: 85-90880

ISBN: 0-449-90188-2

Design by Holly Johnson
Manufactured in the United States of America

First Edition: July 1986

10 9 8 7 6 5 4 3 2 1

Contents

Acknowledgments

I would like to thank the many health professionals who contributed their time and advice in the writing of this book: Ruth Schwartz, M.D.; Anthony Labrum, M.D.; George Trombetta, M.D.; Gwen Sterns, M.D.; Phyllis Collier, R.N.; Sue Greene, R.N.; Michael Kraus; Lucinda Wilcox; Roselle Fine; Mary Beetz; Martha Crawford; and Barbara Conklin. Thanks also to Suzanne Soule, manager of New Life Herbs, for allowing me to consult freely with her on herbal remedies; Laurie Kaiser, of the Women's Career Center, for advice on job reentry; and Elizabeth "Tish" Paddock for access to Planned Parenthood's professional teaching materials. Wendy Wilson, the spunky, warm-hearted founder of Hysterectomy Understanding and Group Support (HUGS) in Rochester, New York, graciously welcomed me to her group's meetings and provided me with important information and leads. Thanks also to Jennifer Fleischer for tips on hair and skin care, and

Edith Nacman, for distributing my menopause questionnaire to her ongoing menopause support group.

Most of all I would like to thank the many women who shared with me their personal experiences with menopause. Their quotes are the real backbone of this book. Thanks also to my writer's support group who cheered me on through the sometimes arduous task of researching and writing. They are: Chloe Barrett, Deborah Raub, Debby Abrahams and Emily Morrison.

I wish to thank the following organizations for sending me research materials: The Center for Climacteric Studies: National Dairy Council; American Institute of Stress; American Academy of Facial, Plastic and Reconstructive Surgery; American Brittle Bone Society; American Cancer Society; American Heart Association; American College of Obstetricians and Gynecologists (a special thanks to Morton Lebow of ACOG—this is the second time he's come through with reams of useful information); Catalyst; Coalition for the Medical Rights of Women; National Institute on Aging; National Mental Health Association; Diamond Headache Clinic; and Santa Fe Health Education Project.

A very special thanks to my editor, Joëlle Delbourgo, whose enthusiastic support made this book possible; and to Michelle Russell, for her helpful editing suggestions. Thanks also are due to Evelyn Podsiadlo, an old friend and editor who got me into this business of book writing in the first place.

Introduction

As a health writer headed toward her middle years, I felt compelled to read about the changes going on within my body. I searched for a good book on menopause. While the market was flooded with literature on pregnancy and child-bearing, I found that little attention had been paid to the needs of older women. Many of the books available were dry and technical, dealing with the problems of menopause and estrogen therapy. This focus on medical problems made menopause sound like some dread disease of the middle-aged.

Menopause is not a shameful ailment of aging women. It does involve some physical and emotional changes. But then, so do puberty and pregnancy—the other major milestones in a woman's reproductive life. After looking at recent statistics I found that the majority of women get through menopause without taking hormones or seeking medical care. In fact, many women who have been through menopause say that it marks a time of renewed self-growth and recharged sexual energy.

I wanted to write a book that would cut through all of the technical terminology, and lead women through the menopause experience in a clear and positive way. It would include all of the traditional medical topics: the physiology of menopause; understanding and coping with hot flashes; the pros and cons of estrogen therapy; body changes at menopause; male and female sexual response in the middle years; and the prevention and treatment of osteoporosis.

I felt it equally important to address the emotional side of menopause—career and role changes, the aging and sometimes death of one's parents, children leaving home, a husband going through mid-life crisis—all of these can take a toll on a woman going through her "changes."

Well-care advice would also be featured, including natural alternatives to estrogen, nutritional needs during menopause, exercise guidelines, dieting tips, stress management techniques and care of aging skin and hair.

It took nearly two years of intensive research to complete *Change of Life*. During that time I corresponded with national women's health groups and major medical organizations, and consulted with experts in many fields—gynecologists, nutritionists, sex counselors, physical education specialists, naturopaths, herbalists, psychologists, career counselors and health educators.

Most importantly of all, I talked to numerous women in all stages of the menopause experience. These women ranged in age from thirty-five to seventy-five. Some were on the threshold of menopause, and beginning to feel the first subtle effects of declining estrogen levels; others were smack dab in the middle of their "changes"; and still others were well past this stage of life.

My subjects included relatives, neighbors, friends and my friends' parents. They were women who exercised with me at the local gym, and senior citizens who attended a local community center. I distributed questionnaires to an ongoing menopause support group sponsored by a family services agency, led a menopause workshop in my living room, and even stopped total strangers at random in public places and asked if they'd be interested in discussing the subject with me. Women referred me to other friends, and so my list grew. I am indebted to these many women. Their personal experiences and helpful advice are interspersed through *Change of Life*.

As you read through *Change of Life* you may find that there are some subjects that you'd like to pursue in more detail. At the end of the book you will find a full list of references for each chapter. I have also compiled a bibliography of suggested readings and addresses of helpful agencies you may want to contact.

Menopause may not be an easy transition for everyone. But it is not so fearful when you understand the events leading up to it, and how to deal with its possible discomforts. My hope is that *Change of Life* will help guide you through menopause in a more confident way.

Chapter 1
What Is
Menopause?
and Other Good
Questions

"My body, in subtle ways, tells me that it's beginning to change. A rush of dizziness now and then, and irregularities in my menstrual cycle made me run to the doctor in a panic. I was told that my problems were hormone-related. That these symptoms were typical for a woman 'of my age.'

"At forty, I still don't think of myself as being middle-aged. I keep trim and active and am doing more things with my life now than I did when the children were babies. I guess my age is sneaking up on me anyway. I've always equated menopause with crazy ladies breaking out in sweats. And worse, with being 'over the hill.' The thought of it depresses me."

"I've heard such scary things about menopause. I've heard that you'll become cranky and irrational and have a diminished sex drive. I'm afraid that I'll become fat and lazy—like an altered cat. It's something I don't want to face. I'll think about it when it happens."

"I've always taken pride in my looks. I wonder how my husband will feel—seeing me with sagging skin and droopy breasts. Will it turn him off? Will he still want me?"

"The childbearing years are a fruit-bearing time. But menopause—it's like becoming a dried-up peach."

Mention the word menopause to women who have not yet gone through it, and chances are you'll see them flinch, joke uncomfortably about it or sigh with resignation. "I know absolutely nothing about it," confesses one forty-one-year-old woman. "I just refuse to believe it's really going to happen to me."

But menopause happens to all healthy and normal women. And the vast majority pass through it beautifully, with only minor complaints. They do not lose their minds or their capacity to enjoy sex. And, if they take good care of themselves, they remain vigorous and attractive.

While menopause is as old as womankind, some dramatic breakthroughs in health care in the past century have put it into an entirely new perspective. It wasn't so long ago that most women died before reaching menopause, or else shortly afterward. A woman living in seventeenth-century Europe had a 28 percent chance of surviving to menopause.[1] By 1900 the female life expectancy in the United States was only forty-eight.[2] It's no wonder that women feared menopause and talked about it in hushed whispers. It was, for them, a sign of declining health and old age.

As a woman today you can expect to live well into your late seventies.[3] That means that you will live a full third of your life *after* menopause. Put another way, you will probably outlive your ovaries by twenty-five to thirty years!

And many women say that the postmenopausal years are some of the best in their lives. Unhampered by child rearing, mothers at last have the time to devote to their own self-fulfillment. With fear of pregnancy past, sexual relationships often bloom anew.

Women entering their middle years today are fortunate in other respects too. They are more open about their bodies and more health conscious than their mothers were. They have been touched by the prepared childbirth movement, the women's movement and by self-help trends in the health field. They are better medical consumers who ask more questions and demand a greater role in their own care.

Since more women than ever before are living past menopause, there is a burgeoning of interest in the subject. Books and articles are beginning to focus on this relatively unexplored area of women's health. But myths and fears that have

Menopause may not be new, but the number of women who are experiencing it is. For the first time in history women can expect to live a full third of their lives after menopause.

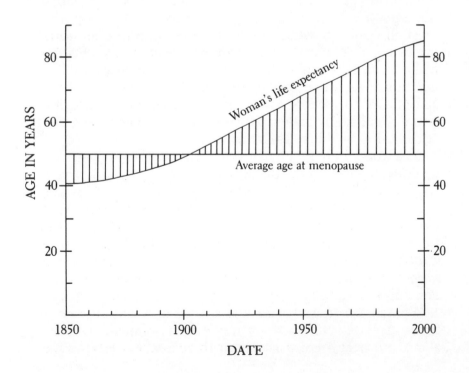

spanned centuries do not die that easily. And you may find that you still have many unanswered questions about the basic facts of menopause.

What Is Menopause?

As you age and become less fertile, you are said to be entering your *climacteric*. The word comes from the Greek, *klimakter*, meaning the step of a staircase or rung of a ladder. It signifies a critical period of life when some important change happens. This image of ascending life's ladder and reaching new heights is fitting for a woman in the prime of her middle years. In medical terms, climacteric is defined as the transitional period between a woman's reproductive life and the end of her fertility.

Sometime during your climacteric your ovaries will stop releasing eggs and you will no longer have periods. The time of your last menstrual period is called *menopause*. You won't know for sure that you have reached menopause until you have gone at least twelve consecutive months without menstruating.

Technically speaking, the years leading up to menopause are called *premenopausal* or *perimenopausal*. The year or two after the final period is defined as *postmenopause*.

Most of us, when talking about menopause, do not make such neat distinctions. In common usage menopause has come to mean any of the changes a woman experiences either before or after she stops menstruating.

At What Age Does Menopause Occur?

A young girl of today can expect to reach puberty at an earlier age than her great-grandmother did. The age of menstrual onset (menarche) has steadily declined in the Western world over the past century. This is probably due to better health care and nutrition. But the average age of menopause has remained about the same—at fifty years—since medieval times. If it has risen at all, it hasn't been by any significant amount.[4,5,6,7]

Most women stop menstruating sometime between the ages

*Menopause occurs during the climacteric. But most people use
these two words interchangeably.*

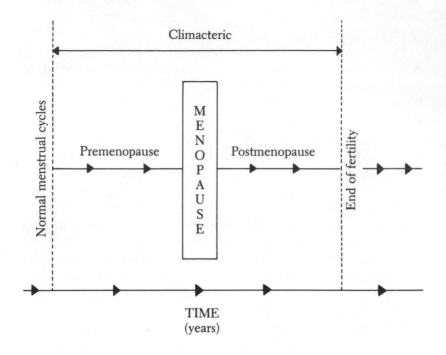

of forty-five and fifty-five, although it is possible for menopause to occur earlier or later than this. Some 10 percent will
cease having periods before their fortieth birthday. This is
considered premature menopause.[8,9]

Why does one woman reach menopause in her forties,
while another menstruates well into her fifties? There are no
clear-cut answers. The age of menopause is a very individual
matter, and each woman seems to have her own inner time
clock.

It was once widely believed that the age of menstrual onset
had some relationship to the age of menopause. Women who
menstruated early supposedly had a late menopause. But this
theory has since been disproven. The age of menopause has

no relationship to the age of menarche, the number of pregnancies, whether or not a woman has breastfed or how old she was when her last pregnancy occurred. Women who are obese may have a slightly later menopause, and unmarried or previously married women may have a slightly earlier one. [10,11]

What about your mother's age at menopause? Can that have any influence on you? Researchers can't seem to agree on this point. However, premature menopause has been observed to run in families. [12,13]

Oddly enough, the only factor definitely known to influence the age of menopause is cigarette smoking. The heavier the smoker, the more likely she is to reach menopause at an earlier age. Exactly what causes this to be so remains a mystery. [14,15]

Artificial menopause can happen at any age. It occurs when a woman's ovaries are removed surgically (oophorectomy) or have been destroyed by radiation or X rays. An artificial menopause is usually abrupt and severe, and a woman must receive hormone treatment for it. If the uterus alone is removed, and one or both ovaries remain, enough hormones are usually produced so that menopause will not occur.

What Are the First Signs?

Nature gives most women some advance notice that menopause is approaching. When you reach your forties, or perhaps even your thirties, you may notice a change in your usual menstrual pattern. These changes can start two, five or even ten or more years before your periods actually come to a halt. Periods may be heavier than usual or much lighter. They may come closer together or further apart. Some women's cycles seem to go haywire: a heavy flow one month, followed by a light staining the next; or a twenty-three-day cycle followed by one that is fifty days long.

In the year or two before menopause, periods usually become scantier and further apart until they cease altogether. However, menopause may also come without warning. Some women menstruate regularly right up until their final period.

When it comes to menopause, the exception is the rule. Every woman seems to have a unique story to tell.

"The first thing I noticed was a change in my periods. They were always regular before. Now they were becoming heavy and irregular. Some months they would last seven days instead of my usual five. Other months they would last four days. This went on for several years, until I began missing periods altogether. I'd have all of the premenstrual symptoms but no release. The last year was really bad. I'd skip my periods for a few months and then I'd get cramps and backaches when I did get them—with a heavy flow. Then all of a sudden they stopped. The whole process took five or six years."

"I'm forty-nine years old, and my doctor has considered me premenopausal for the past ten years. That's when my periods started to change. I used to begin my period slowly, and by the third day I was in full bloom, and had very bad cramps. Now I start off with a bang and taper off, sometimes crampy and sometimes not. I still menstruate every twenty-eight days, but my periods can last three days one month, and then sometimes eight or nine the next."

"I always got my periods like clockwork for six or seven days. It was very heavy the first two days. I'd have to race to the bathroom. Then, when I turned fifty, my periods just stopped. I never had a symptom."

"My family goes through early menopause. My mother at forty-one, my aunt in her late thirties. I'm only thirty-two, but I've been having attacks of dizziness and my period is becoming irregular and very heavy. My mother had the same thing. She had one D & C (dilation and curettage) after another. They never found anything wrong. I'm resigning myself to the same thing."

"Soon after I turned forty my periods became occasionally late or early. They don't last as long as they used to, and they're very light—sometimes a stain instead of a flow. I asked my doctor if this could possibly be the beginning of menopause, but he just shrugged and said, 'maybe.'"

Your periods may stop for reasons other than menopause.

Severe emotional stress, an accident or illness may hold menstruation at bay. One woman who nearly died of encephalitis when she was in her thirties reports that her periods stopped for four years. After a series of tests her doctor diagnosed her as having a premature menopause. Then, "as if out of the blue" she says, her periods started again at the age of forty-one. Everything else appeared to be normal and her doctor was "simply flabbergasted."

There is one other good reason why your periods may stop, and that is pregnancy. As long as you are menstruating—be it six or even two times a year—it is possible for you to conceive. Since menopause can only be recognized by hindsight, it is recommended that women who use contraceptives continue doing so for at least one full year following their last menstrual period. Some authorities even recommend that you do so for two years.[16]

Are There Any Other Symptoms?

Menopause used to be a convenient scapegoat for the medical world. Virtually every middle-age female health complaint was blamed on "the changes." According to one article in the *Journal of Nurse Midwifery*, in the year 1880, 135 different symptoms were attributed to menopause, including "hysterical flatulance" and "temporary deafness."[17]

Today, most medical experts will tell you that only three symptoms result directly from a decrease in female hormone levels:[18] (1) Hot flashes or flushes—sudden surges of warmth in the face, neck and chest. When they occur at night, they are called "night sweats." (2) A loss of moisture and elasticity in the vagina, described medically as "vaginal atrophy." (Women with active sex lives or who masturbate regularly are less troubled by this.) (3) Loss of bone density. Sometime around the age of thirty-five a woman's bones begin to lose calcium. For the majority of women this poses no problems. However, one out of four will develop osteoporosis, a bone disease that leaves women vulnerable to increased fractures in later life.

Other common discomforts reported by women around the time of menopause include: headache, fatigue, dizziness, insomnia, mood swings, palpitations, tingling in fingers and toes, shortness of breath, weight gain, aching joints, nervousness and irritability. Physicians disagree as to whether these symptoms are the result of changing hormone levels, or whether they stem from emotional stresses which usually accompany the middle years.

Most women will experience some of these discomforts during menopause—but few will experience *all* of them. In one study nearly 16 percent of women had no symptoms at all.[19]

Menopausal problems are usually short-lived, lasting an average of two to five years. They are temporary and normal, and not a sign of illness. Learning what to expect can help you to deal with them more calmly. A more detailed look at each of these symptoms and how to cope with them is presented in a later chapter.

How Severe Will Your Symptoms Be?

In most cases, menopause is a gradual process which causes moderate discomfort. Studies have shown that 75 to 85 percent of all women are not troubled enough by symptoms to seek medical assistance.[20]

How severe your symptoms will be probably depends upon how quickly your hormone levels drop, as well as on your individual sensitivity to hormonal changes. When hormone levels plummet, there is little time for the body to adjust. This is what happens after a hysterectomy if both ovaries have been removed. The sudden withdrawal of estrogen can cause very severe flushes and painful vaginal dryness. Hormone therapy is usually necessary to relieve these symptoms.

A small number of women seem especially sensitive to hormonal fluctuations. A woman who has suffered from premenstrual tension and postpartum depression may tend to have severe menopausal symptoms too.[21]

Your mental outlook can also play a part. The person whose life is humming along smoothly, and who has satisfying work and supportive personal relationships may take hot flushes and the aches and pains of menopause in her stride. But the woman who feels disoriented by the empty-nest syndrome, and has marital difficulties or problems with ailing parents or a particularly stressful job may not cope as well. To her, menopause may seem like the proverbial straw that broke the camel's back.

A good marriage, fulfilling work and a stimulating environment have all been shown to ease the stresses of menopause.[22,23] This does not mean that happily married career women don't have hot flushes, headaches or vaginal dryness. It simply means that those who keep busy and have emotional support at home will probably concentrate less on their physical discomforts.

Will You Become Depressed or Lose Your Mind?

No, your mind will not turn to mush when your ovaries stop functioning. This is an old wives' tale grown out of the fact that severe mental illness in older women was, at one time, diagnosed as involutional melancholia—a mental illness of the middle years. In truth, there is no more evidence of severe depression among women at this time of their lives than at any other.[24,25]

In a frequently cited 1964 study, sociologist Bernice Neugarten presented 460 women aged thirteen to sixty-four with a checklist of twenty-eight symptoms generally attributed to menopause. She found that it was the adolescents—and *not* the middle-aged women in the group—who reported having the most emotional symptoms. Women going through menopause reported having more physical symptoms. And women finished with menopause checked off the fewest symptoms of all.[26]

Another researcher found that when menopause occurred unusually early or late it was more likely to trigger psychological distress. When menopause occurred at its expected time there were no unusual emotional problems.[27]

Many women feel saddened by the loss of menstrual cycles, though if you ask them, they do not really find the thought of bearing and raising another baby either practical or appealing at this stage of the game.

"I don't mind not having the mess of menstruating or the bother of coping with contraceptives, but I've grown used to

being a cyclical person—to the familiarity of my body at different times of the month. When I'm cross and irritable my husband always jokes about it—'Oh, you must be getting your period.' And I get to pamper myself at that time of the month. I could really get a lot of mileage out of my period from my family when I wanted to use it as an excuse."

"At age forty-seven the last thing I would want right now is to have more children. I am looking forward to devoting more time to me for a change. Still, there is a certain sadness about leaving the mothering part of me behind."

"Not having periods any more is like moving from a climate where there are many different seasons to one that is warm all of the time. I will probably enjoy the rows of sunny days, without the bleeding and bloating and mood swings, but I'm going to miss the changing seasons too."

For most women, menopause is a time for reflection and for a wistful glance backwards. It marks the end of an important era in your life. You may feel liberated and saddened at the same time—a bittersweet mixture. But then, as one woman matter-of-factly says, "you simply get on with it."

Will You Become Less Attractive or Desirable?

There is no reason why a woman would become less feminine or sexually attractive following menopause. To prove this to yourself just look around you. Think about all of the sharp and sexy middle-aged women on stage and screen, in politics and in your own community. You certainly wouldn't describe actresses Linda Evans, Joan Collins and Sophia Loren as being "over-the-hill." Tina Turner continues to "turn on" ever-younger generations of rock music fans. And women's activists Jane Fonda and Gloria Steinem show that brains and beauty do indeed flourish in women in their forties and fifties. You undoubtedly know many outstanding middle-aged women in your own personal life too. They are substantial people who exude a self-confidence that a younger, less mature woman doesn't have.

True, we are all aging from the day of birth. As you reach your middle years you no longer have the supple skin or taut muscles of youth. But that doesn't mean that you are no longer attractive. With good nutrition and regular exercise you can stay trim and vigorous looking. Women who take care of themselves, who are physically and mentally active and have a positive self-image, are attractive to everyone all of their lives.

If you and your mate have a good sexual relationship, you are likely to continue to enjoy this facet of your lives after menopause. An active sex life is beneficial to you—it helps to maintain vaginal lubrication and elasticity. If you do run into problems with vaginal dryness, there are ways to cope, and these will be discussed elsewhere in this book.

Although it sometimes takes more time to respond sexually as we grow older, most men and women continue to desire and enjoy sexual relations well into old age.[78] Some women report that they are more interested in sex following their menopause. The added years help many to shed inhibitions—to experiment more and to tell their partners what pleases them. Gone is the fear of pregnancy, and freedom from contraception and children around the house can mean more spontaneous lovemaking. "With our children grown and out of the house," says one woman, "it feels like a second honeymoon."

Experience also brings understanding. You are able to be more sensitive to your mate and to his needs. The added years have most likely made you a better, more considerate lover.

A Time for Personal Growth

You hear a lot about the problems of menopause, but hardly anyone goes around trumpeting the good news—and that is, menopause ushers in an exciting time of personal freedom and growth.

It is often younger women who paint unrealistically drab pictures of what it is like to be menopausal. In one landmark study, the attitudes of women who had not yet gone through menopause were compared with those of women who had. The most negative feelings about menopause came from the younger women. Middle-aged women described a "recovery" following menopause and even some "marked gains" once menopause was past. Postmenopausal women saw themselves as "feeling better, more confident, calmer, freer than before."[29]

With children grown, and the responsibilities of rearing a young family over, many middle-aged women are at last free to pay attention to their own interests. They may take up new hobbies, or even new careers, with an enthusiasm unparalleled since they were in their teens. Anthropologist Margaret Mead noticed this infusion of energy in the middle years. She labeled the phenomenon PMZ—short for postmenopausal zest.[30]

"Perhaps with education and proper perspective, we can look forward to the day when people will stop viewing menopause as a crisis, or even as 'the change,' and see it more appropriately as 'yet another change,'" writes Dr. Kathryn E. McGoldrick, editor of the *Journal of the American Medical Women's Association.* "For living is constant change. That is its essence and its promise."[31]

Chapter 2
The
Female
Hormones

Your body does not shut off its supply of female hormones like a faucet in one day. Menopause is the end result of a very gradual process which began when you were in your mid-twenties. It takes several decades for hormone levels to decrease to the point where menstruation is no longer possible. And even when you no longer have periods, your body continues to supply you with small amounts of female hormones. To put menopause into its proper perspective it is helpful to take a step backwards and look at the changing role of female hormones throughout a woman's life span.

The word hormone comes from the Greek "to stimulate." And that is what hormones do. They are chemical messengers. Produced in one part of the body, they course through the bloodstream to another part, prodding it to take some kind of action.

Hormones are produced in the endocrine glands. Secretions from these glands orchestrate male and female sexual

Changes in Estrogen Levels as a Woman Ages

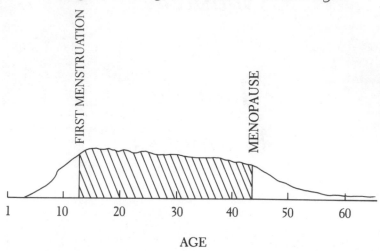

AGE

development at puberty, and control all facets of our daily lives. Men and women have the exact same endocrine glands, but with two notable exceptions: the female ovaries and the male testes. These are also called the sex glands or gonads.

The ovaries are two walnut-shaped bodies located on either side of your uterus. They are small glands—weighing under two ounces[1]—but they pack a powerful hormonal wallop. During the childbearing years the ovaries busily manufacture large quantities of estrogen and progesterone. These two powerful sex hormones govern the monthly menstrual cycles. When their cyclic release is disturbed, as it is in the years before menopause, a woman may experience menstrual irregularities.

From Birth to Puberty: The Awakening of Female Sexuality

A newborn female is born with all of the equipment she will need for reproduction. Inside her miniature ovaries are stored all of the eggs she will ever produce in her lifetime. Nature has, in fact, been overbounteous with her initial supply of ova. There are approximately 500,000 of them within the ovaries at birth, though only 400 to 500 of these will ever fully ripen and be released during the menstrual cycle.[2] The rest of the eggs degenerate over the years until only a few are left at the time of menopause.

If you looked at one of the egg cells under a microscope you would see that it is actually an immature egg nestled within a protective ball of cells. Together, egg and surrounding cells are called a Graafian follicle, described first by the seventeenth-century Dutch scientist Regnier de Graaf.

The period from birth to adolescence is a very quiet one with regard to female hormonal activity. Once in a while, an infant girl will have a bloody discharge from her vagina immediately after birth. In such rare cases the baby is excreting excess hormones she received from her mother in the latter stages of pregnancy. For the most part, however, female hormone production is negligible until a girl reaches puberty.

Then, somewhere between the ages of ten and thirteen, an internal alarm clock goes off. The brain directs the ovaries to secrete increasing amounts of the female hormone estrogen into the girl's bloodstream. Scientists believe that the time of this biological alarm is determined by a girl's weight and fat composition; they must rise to a certain critical level before estrogen can be released into her system. This may be nature's way of assuring that a young woman has enough calories stored within her body to meet the demands of pregnancy and lactation.[3,4]

As estrogen floods into her bloodstream, a girl blossoms. Her breasts develop, pubic and underarm hair grows, the uterus, ovaries and vagina mature, and a new layer of fat gives her feminine curves and the rounded hips of a woman. Finally, she gets her first menstrual period.

The Menstrual Cycle

The study of hormones began only fifty years ago.[5] And it is only since the 1960s and early '70s that scientists began to unravel the complex dynamics of the menstrual cycle.[6] They have learned that a woman's monthly cycles are based upon a delicate feedback system. The hypothalamus, pituitary gland and ovaries send hormonal messages back and forth to each other, influencing each other's actions.

The events of the menstrual cycle can be difficult to follow, especially if you are unfamiliar with the terminology. As you read through the following material you may find it helpful to consult the glossary of menstrual terms on page 30.

Step One: *The Hypothalamus Switches the Menstrual Cycle "On"*

The hypothalamus, a small area of specialized brain cells above the pituitary gland, can be likened to a power switch. Each month it turns the menstrual cycle "on" by sending a chemical message to the pituitary gland.

Step Two: *The Pituitary Sends Two Hormones to the Ovaries*

Next the pituitary, the so-called "master gland" at the base of the brain, takes over the show. It begins by secreting two hormones into the bloodstream: FSH (follicle-stimulating hormone) and LH (luteinizing hormone). FSH and LH are called gonadotropic hormones because they are aimed, like arrows, directly at the gonads or ovaries.

Step Three: *Estrogen Levels Rise and Peak*

Follicle-stimulating hormone does what its name implies: when it reaches the ovaries it stimulates eight or nine of the Graafian follicles to swell and develop. At the same time it causes the uterine lining to begin thickening in preparation for a possible pregnancy. At the beginning of the menstrual cycle, FSH is queen and this stage is called the follicular phase.

As the follicles mature, they in turn release a hormone of their own: estrogen. The amount of estrogen in the blood begins to build, finally reaching a crescendo. At this point, the pituitary gets the message that too much estrogen is present in the bloodstream. To lower the rising volume of estrogen, the pituitary cuts back on FSH production and releases a new surge of LH.

The Menstrual System

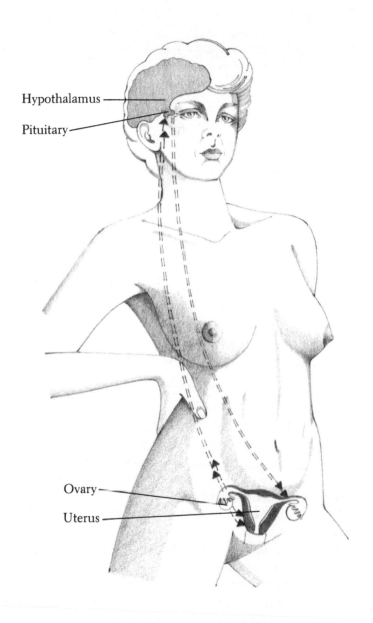

Hypothalamus

Pituitary

Ovary

Uterus

Hormonal Fluctuations Throughout the Menstrual Cycle

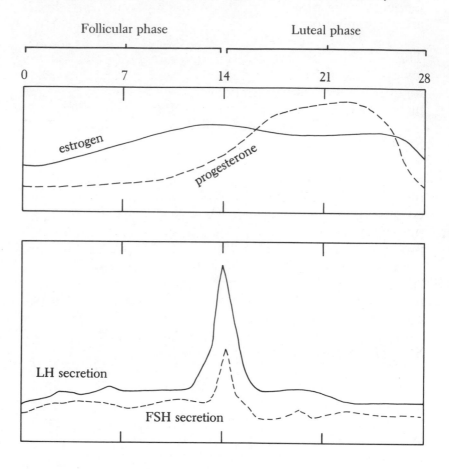

Step Four: Ovulation Takes Place

Now luteinizing hormone takes central stage in the menstrual drama. And this part of the cycle is known as the luteal phase. When LH gets to the ovaries it singles out one of the maturing follicles and fully ripens it. This completely matured follicle moves to the ovarian wall, where it bursts open, releasing the egg inside. The egg begins its journey down the fallopian tube. In the meantime, the other partially developed follicles degenerate.

This bursting of the egg from its sac is called ovulation. It usually occurs fourteen days before a woman gets her period. Conception is possible within twelve to twenty-four hours after ovulation occurs.

Some women know the exact time that they are ovulating. They can feel the egg bursting out as a sharp pain on the lower left or right side of their abdomen. The medical term for this is mittelschmerz (middle pain). A woman may also have a light staining during the time of ovulation.

Step Five: Progesterone Thickens the Uterine Lining

Everything seems to have a purpose in nature and even the used sac, now empty of its egg, plays an important role in the menstrual cycle. It turns a yellowish color and becomes the corpus luteum (meaning yellow body). The newly formed corpus luteum produces estrogen, plus a new hormone— progesterone.

Progesterone is the hormone of pregnancy. Its name means "pro-gestation" or "in favor of pregnancy." This hormone makes the uterine lining even thicker and spongier: a hospitable place for a fertilized egg to nest.

Step Six: Menstruation Occurs

If the egg is fertilized the corpus luteum continues to secrete estrogen and progesterone until the growing placenta can take over its job. When fertilization does not occur, the corpus luteum dies, and estrogen and progesterone levels fall. With its main source of nourishment cut off, the uterine lining is sloughed off in what is known as menstruation.

Step Seven: The Cycle Starts Anew

Events now come full circle. The hypothalamus, alerted by the body's lowered state of estrogen, sets into action once more. It instructs the pituitary to begin sending out FSH and LH. And so the intricate dance of hormones begins once more.

Cycle Changes Before Menopause

All animals appear to experience waning fertility as they age. But unlike humans, most other female mammals ovulate,

The Menstrual Cycle

Day 5

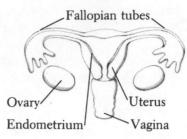

Fallopian tubes

Ovary

Endometrium

Uterus

Vagina

Day 14 (ovulation)

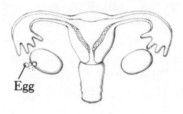

Egg

Day 19

Egg

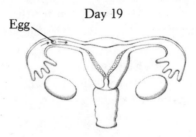

Day 1 of new cycle

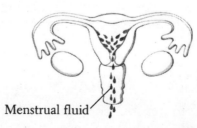

Menstrual fluid

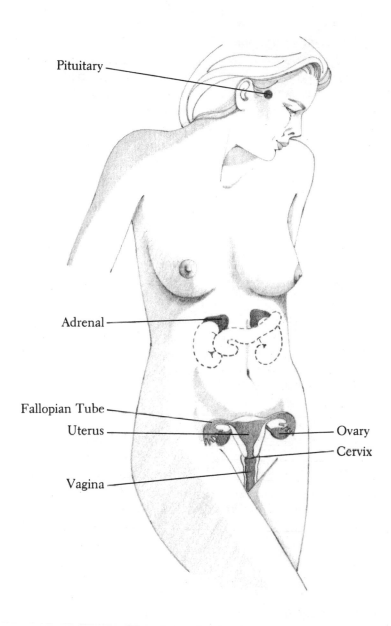

Pituitary

Adrenal

Fallopian Tube

Uterus

Ovary

Cervix

Vagina

Female Reproductive Anatomy: Endocrine Glands and Sexual Organs

even if sporadically, almost until the very end of their lives. Human beings spend a sizable chunk of their life span—about twenty-five to thirty years—in a fully nonreproductive state. This may be because human babies have a prolonged need for nurturing. A woman needs to be around long after menopause to see her youngest offspring safely to maturity.[7,8]

No one knows exactly why all of the changes of menopause come about. But somewhere along the way the delicate feedback system between hypothalamus, pituitary and ovaries is interrupted. Signals between the body's messengers become confused, and the glands frantically secrete too little or too much hormone in an effort to set things straight.

As you approach your final menstrual period your stock of egg cells is almost entirely used up, and the Graafian follicles that do remain are not as responsive to hormonal stimulation as they used to be. These follicles mature in a hit-or-miss fashion. Some months they can be aroused enough by FSH to ripen and release an egg, other months they cannot. This means that estrogen and progesterone levels vary widely from month to month, resulting in menstrual irregularities.

In the year or two before menopause most of a woman's cycles become anovulatory—that is, without the release of eggs. Menstrual periods tend to come at increasingly longer intervals. Finally, the follicles no longer respond at all. Estrogen levels drop. Progesterone is no longer produced. And menstruation occurs no more.

This is all as it should be. The purpose of the menstrual cycle, remember, is for a woman to be able to conceive and bear a child. After a reproductive life span that lasts approximately thirty-five years the ovaries have finished their work. This comes at a time in a woman's life when it is no longer physically or emotionally desirable for her to have any more babies.

The Hormones After Menopause

The hypothalamus and pituitary seem at first oblivious to the fact that menopause has occurred. They act as if there were still healthy follicles in the ovaries. After receiving its customary signal from the hypothalamus, the pituitary continues to send out FSH and LH. Only now, when FSH arrives at the ovaries, nothing happens. The few remaining follicles are incapable of ripening.

In a valiant, but fruitless effort to rescue these degenerated egg cells, the pituitary floods the bloodstream with massive doses of FSH. In fact, FSH levels in menopausal women rise from five to twenty times their normal amount. LH levels rise too, reaching from three to five times their normal level.[9,10] This same surge of FSH and LH is experienced by women who have had their ovaries removed, usually within two to three days after surgery.[11]

FSH and LH levels are at their highest at about two or three years following menopause. They will decline very gradually over the next thirty years, until they are at about half of the menopausal level.[12]

A Continuous Supply of Estrogen

Estrogen production declines dramatically after menopause, but it never stops altogether. The body is a cleverly devised machine. Once the ovaries stop functioning at full tilt, other glands and body cells pitch in to help provide some of the missing hormone.

The fat cells in a woman's body play a major role in the production of estrogen after menopause. Like the fabled alchemist who could turn lead into gold, the fat tissue can take androgens (male hormones) and convert them into estrone, a weak form of estrogen.

Small amounts of male hormones circulate within a woman's body throughout the childbearing years. They are produced in the ovaries and the adrenals, two glands located on top of your kidneys. After menopause, the ovaries continue to secrete a small amount of male hormones, but it is the adrenal glands that contribute the bulk of the supply.

The amount of estrone in a postmenopausal woman's body seems to be influenced by her weight. The heavier a woman is, and the higher the percentage of body fat, the more likely she is to have high levels of estrone in her bloodstream. Thus, obese women tend to have less severe menopausal symptoms than their thinner sisters.[13,14,15]

Conversion of Male Hormones to Estrogen in the Body's Fat Tissues

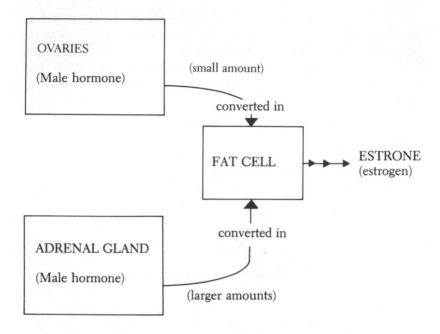

There is much individual variation in the amount of estrone a woman will produce after menopause. Though it's certainly not the rule, some women maintain estrogen levels that are as high or higher than they were before menopause.[16] This is probably true of those who sail through their menopause without any symptoms or discomforts.

Though estrogen is being produced by the body, it is no longer released cyclically as it was during the menstrual years. Instead, the body produces it in a stable, steady fashion.

Male Menopause

Do men have a menopause too? The answer is an unequivocal no. A woman is born with all of the eggs she will ever produce in her lifetime. At menopause, the supply becomes depleted, and she becomes completely infertile. A man, on the other hand, can produce a new supply of sperm every time he ejaculates. He is capable of fathering children in his seventies, eighties and even nineties![17] (The oldest woman on record to have successfully completed a pregnancy was fifty-seven years and 129 days old.)[18]

There is nothing in the male experience to compare with the profound hormonal changes at menopause. The term "male menopause" which has been bandied about refers only to the emotional changes a man faces in his middle years. A normal, sexually active male will experience a very gradual decrease in his fertility with age, but the changes are never as tumultuous or complete as they are for a woman.[19]

Parallels with Puberty

It was natural for your periods to begin at puberty and it is equally natural that they stop at menopause. These two transitional periods are biological opposites, one a gearing up of the reproductive system, the other a winding down process.

At puberty, a girl's estrogen levels are still low, and even though she is menstruating, her cycles are not fully fertile. Some months her ovaries fail to release a mature egg. And for the first year or two she is likely to experience menstrual irregularities and skip a cycle here and there.[20]

A very similar situation exists at menopause. As estrogen levels taper off you occasionally fail to ovulate. Menstrual cycles become erratic. And though it is still possible for you to become pregnant you are not as fertile as you were before.

Unlike the adolescent, however, you have the advantage of your experience to fall back on. Over the years women grow used to upheavals in their body's chemistry—to the rhythmic swell and fall of the menstrual cycles, and to the extraordinary changes of pregnancy and lactation. They learn to adapt to changing roles, from young woman to wife to mother. A woman who has learned to weather so many changes is likely to come to grips with this new transition in a mature and confident way.

A Menstrual Cycle Glossary

Corpus Luteum: A yellow body formed when the egg bursts out of its protective sac. The empty sac, or corpus luteum, produces estrogen and progesterone, which nourish the uterine lining. After menopause no corpus luteum is formed, and therefore no progesterone is secreted.

Estrogen: Secreted by the ovaries. The most powerful of female hormones. Estrogen causes a girl to develop into womanhood. Declining levels lead to menopause and play a part in menopausal flushes and vaginal dryness. Following menopause, estrogen is produced mainly by conversion of male hormones, or androgens, to estrone. This conversion takes place in the body's fat cells.

Follicle-Stimulating Hormone (FSH): Secreted by the pituitary. FSH stimulates the development of eight or nine follicles within the ovaries each month. It also makes the uterine lining start to thicken. FSH levels may increase up to twenty-fold after menopause.

Follicular Phase: The initial phase of the menstrual cycle leading up to ovulation, also known as the proliferative phase. It varies in length from woman to woman and cycle to cycle. Before menopause a shortened follicular phase may cause periods to be spaced more closely together.

Graafian Follicle: The egg and its surrounding ball of cells.

Hypothalamus: A small area of the brain above the pituitary. It "kicks off" the menstrual cycle by sending a chemical message to the pituitary gland.

Luteal Phase: (Also referred to as the secretory phase.) This is the second phase of the menstrual period. It is marked by ovulation and a thickening of the uterine lining. It usually lasts from twelve to fourteen days. During this phase conception is possible.

Luteinizing Hormone (LH): A pituitary hormone that selects and fully ripens one egg per month (though occasionally more than one may be ripened at the same time). LH causes the egg to burst from its sac and makes the uterine lining increasingly thick and spongy. After menopause LH levels rise three- to fivefold.

Pituitary: A pea-size gland at the base of the brain. Called the "master gland" because it has control over so many other endocrine glands. At a signal from the hypothalamus it sends out varying amounts of FSH and LH—two hormones which profoundly affect events within the ovaries.

Progesterone: The hormone that thickens the uterus in preparation for pregnancy. It is produced by the corpus luteum. During the premenopausal stage a lack of progesterone can cause incomplete shedding of the uterus and heavy periods. After menopause the corpus luteum fails to form and progesterone is no longer produced.

Chapter 3
Hot
Flashes

"*My first experience of flashes was when my mother's cronies came over to play bridge. All night long the window of our tiny kitchen would fly up and down as first one, and then another got a hot flash. They giggled over it, and teased each other. Now I'm going through it. But I don't see so much to laugh about.*"

Hot flashes are the classic sign of menopause. An estimated 75 to 85 percent of women experience them to some degree.[1,2,3] For some, they begin during the premenopausal years when the length and flow of the menstrual cycles begin to change. Others don't experience their first hot flash until after they have had their final menstrual period. Hot flashes are harmless and temporary, usually occurring over a period of from one to five years. But they can be a nuisance and a source of embarrassment. Only a relatively small number of women (10 to 15 percent) find that their flashes are severe enough to warrant medical treatment.[4,5]

What's Happening to Me?

When they first occur, hot flashes may take you by surprise. You may blame everything from illness to a faulty air-conditioning system before realizing what the source of your personal heat wave really is.

"It was a summer evening and my husband and I were out having dinner with friends. We were chatting and drinking cocktails when all of a sudden my body felt flushed with heat. Sweat came pouring off of my face. I felt as if I wanted to tear off my clothes. 'We'd better go home,' I said to my husband. 'I think I've got a case of the summer flu.'"

"I am normally a warm person, always perspiring easily and needing the windows open at home and work. In fact, I used to kid around and say I'd never know it when a real hot flash came. I had just been to the doctor for a checkup and he told me that my blood pressure was a little high. Soon after I noticed that my face periodically got all hot and red and that I would perspire profusely. I was in the faculty room at school when it happened to me again. I commented to a colleague, 'I'm so worried, I think my blood pressure must be going up.' She said, 'It looks more to me like you're having hot flashes. I've been noticing that you've been having them for weeks.' I was tremendously relieved and grateful to her for telling me that."

"I had just moved to Washington, D.C. The summers were hotter than I was used to. So when I began to have hot flashes I blamed it on the weather. I even went out and got my hair cut really short, foolishly thinking that it would cool me off."

Since flashes can, in some instances, be a sign of illness, it may be a good idea to mention them to your doctor when they first occur. However, if your periods are becoming irregular or have stopped for several months and you are in your forties or fifties, chances are that your suspected hot flashes are just that.

What It Feels Like

Most everyone is familiar with the sight of a menopausal woman experiencing a hot flash. She's the one who complains of the heat while everyone else around her seems perfectly comfortable. She may throw off her sweater, fan herself frantically and open windows in an effort to cool off. Then, just as abruptly, she begins to shiver and searches for the sweater she discarded minutes before. These shifts from hot to cold may seem comical or puzzling to others. But for the woman herself they are just plain annoying.

Most hot flashes start as a sudden and overwhelming sensation of warmth on the face, upper chest and neck. The heat usually spreads upward or downward in waves, and a woman's face and chest may become splotchy or bright red. Perspiration sometimes forms on the face, head, neck and back. When the heat wave subsides, a woman is usually left with a chilled, clammy feeling. The entire episode is usually over within two or three minutes. In rarer instances it may go on for as long as half an hour or more.

While this is a typical description of a hot flash, there is plenty of room for individual variation. No two women seem to experience a flash in exactly the same way. And the same woman may have a different experience from one flash episode to another.

A flash can be so mild and fleeting that a woman is unsure whether or not she is experiencing one. Or it can make your entire body feel as if it's on fire, and leave profuse perspiration in its wake. They may come as often as every ten minutes, or as infrequently as once a month. Most flashes fall somewhere in between these possible extremes. When a woman is still menstruating she may find that her flashes start out mild and increase in number and intensity following her final menstrual period.

The highly unpredictable nature of hot flashes was confirmed in a study of twenty women who had a total of 1,041 hot flashes over a two-week period. The investigator found that these flashes varied in intensity and that they could begin anywhere on the body and spread in different directions. [6,7]

Many people use the words hot flash and hot flush to mean the same thing, but this is not entirely accurate. A flash refers to all of the sensations a woman feels, while a flush refers only to the reddening of the skin. Not everyone who has a hot flash experiences flushing.

Warning Signals

For some, flashes come suddenly, without any advance warning. Others describe an unusual sensation that builds within them before the actual flash begins. It may feel like pressure in the head or like a heightening nervousness or anxiety.

"Right before a flash I can feel my body tense up. I get rigid. I feel like screaming. I have to hold myself together and tell myself that this feeling will pass."

"I feel the blood rushing to my head and I think I am going to faint. My heart beats very hard. When it happens I really get scared."

Night Sweats

When hot flashes occur at night they're called "night sweats." A woman who has them may wake up sopping wet and have to change her night clothes and bed linens, or she may merely feel slightly warm, needing only to kick off her covers for relief. Not everyone who has hot flashes gets them at night. However, those who have night sweats always have hot flashes during the day as well. As with daytime flashes, they occur in no set pattern. Some women get them several times each night while others experience them only once in a while.

How troublesome night flashes are depends a lot upon how easily you are able to return to sleep after a disturbance. One woman says that she can get up, change her nightgown and go back to sleep again as soon as her head hits the pillow. Others find it next to impossible to settle down again. If this is true in your case you may want to refer to the discussion on insomnia presented in the next chapter.

Physical Symptoms That May Accompany Flashes

Some women note a feeling of suffocation or shortness of breath when they are having a flash. They may also experience one or more of the following: palpitations, nausea, weakness, fatigue, dizziness, headaches, formication (a feeling that insects are crawling across your skin) and numbness or tingling in the fingers or toes. These symptoms are most likely related to the hormonal havoc that is going on as your body adjusts to lowered levels of estrogen, but they can also be signs of emotional distress or of other potentially serious circulatory problems. It's important that you report them to your physician.

Palpitations are probably the most alarming symptom. A woman's heart may pound so violently that she is sure she is having a heart attack.

"I sometimes get palpitations at night. It's a feeling of my heart beating and blood rushing through my veins. It doesn't happen every time I get a flash. The first time it happened I thought I was dying. The doctor asked if I wanted a tranquilizer. I said no. Now that I know it's normal I won't be frightened and I can relax."

"I can actually feel my pulse beating through my side or my back as I lie in bed or sit in a chair. I don't do anything special for it, aside from trying to relax. There's never any pain."

"First a feeling of weakness passes over me and then the palpitations come. My heart pounds so loud it frightens me. I asked my husband if he could hear it too, but he said no. The doctor doesn't seem to think anything of it. While I'm having them it helps if I take a very deep breath."

If you experience palpitations with hot flashes it is probably nothing to worry about. You should of course consult with your doctor to rule out circulatory problems. And you might also benefit by cutting down or eliminating stimulants such as coffee, tea, tobacco, caffeinated soft drinks and chocolate.

Emotional Symptoms

Around the time of menopause, many women also complain of mood swings, fatigue, irritability and anxiety. These may well be due to emotional stress, as many physicians believe. But they may also be indirectly caused by hot flashes. Explains one doctor: "If you were sitting peacefully in a room and I came and shoved you, what would happen? Your heart rate would probably speed up, and you'd become emotional. If I did it to you again and again throughout the day, you would undoubtedly become irritable. Think of a flash in the same way. A woman's equilibrium is being disturbed over and over again. What's more, she has no idea when all of this will end."

Night sweats can also contribute to emotional symptoms. The woman whose sleep is disturbed night after night will undoubtedly feel wrung out, irritable and moody during the day.

Things That Can Set a Hot Flash Off

Hot flashes may seem to come out of the blue. But often they are triggered by outside stimuli. Anything that raises your temperature may set off a flash. Emotions such as anxiety, nervousness, anger or sexual excitement can do it. So can alcohol, warm drinks, hot weather, being in a crowded room or simply getting under the bedcovers.[8]

One investigator noted that his subject had a special sensitivity to sounds, particularly during the early evening hours. She was likely to flash at the sound of a doorbell, telephone or a person suddenly talking.[9]

"I notice my flashes most when I am completely at rest and feeling relaxed," observes one woman. She inevitably gets one when she attends her subscription performance to the symphony and, oddly enough, when she's at home ironing. "I like ironing. I'm probably one of the only women who still irons her husband's shirts, even though they're wash and wear. I find it relaxing. I cradle the phone against one ear so I can chat with a friend and iron at the same time. I always draw the drapes first. I just know I'll be taking my T-shirt off and on at least three or four times within the hour."

If you write down the conditions during which you usually have a hot flash you may see your own pattern appear. Perhaps you can avoid the situations that are likely to trigger a flash, or at least be prepared for their likely occurrence.

Personal Stories

It's impossible to predict whether or not a woman will have hot flashes, or if she does, how mild or severe they may be. An informal survey reveals a wide range of personal experiences.

"One of my co-workers had the hot flashes terribly. She said to me, 'Wait until you have to go through it.' I was horrified at the thought. But when I got the flashes they were really very mild. They lasted two years and then were over. I guess everyone is different, and you can't let other people's stories frighten you."—Age fifty-four.

"I had a severe case, probably tied up to emotional problems (I lost my husband around that time). I had hot flashes every ten minutes and violent palpitations. I felt like my body was on fire. It started at the bottom of my legs and travelled up to my head. My hair would be dripping. My kids would say, 'Mom, you're having a flash.' Over the past three years my flashes are getting fewer and fewer. Now they come once an hour, or even less. They're nowhere as intense as before. My mom had flashes until she was in her seventies."—Age fifty-two.

"I get warm, but not soaked. Sometimes I'm not even sure if I'm really having one or not. Occasionally, I'm a little warm in the middle of the night. By nature I'm always cold—with icy feet and hands—so this is new to me."—Age fifty-five.

"I can just be sitting there and it happens all of a sudden. The heat rises from my neck up, but never involves any other part of my body. I never feel dizzy or have any palpitations. For three years I had them about ten times a day. I would wake up nights and unconsciously pull my covers off and then pull them back on again five minutes later. Insomnia was never any problem. The flashes seemed to come in cycles. I sometimes went weeks without having any flashes at all, and then I'd get them ten times a day for a few days in a row. It was just uncomfortable, but really no great bother. I'm almost completely through with them now. I still get one occasionally.— Age fifty-five.

"My story is a very peculiar one, I'm sure. I don't know anyone else who has it like me. When I was fifty my periods stopped and I had no other symptoms. Then ten years later I started to have the flashes. I'd be at work and suddenly my blood would feel as if it were rushing to my head and a feeling of weakness came over me. I also got palpitations. I still get flashes once in a while, mainly when I'm tense. I used to have the flashes several times a month, but now it might happen once and not again for three months."—Age sixty-eight.

"For me flashes don't come in waves. I get warmer and warmer until my cheeks burn and turn a brilliant red. Sometimes my heart pounds. At the time it's embarrassing. People at work look at me and know I'm having one. I think the flashes occur more premenstrually—a week to ten days before I get my period. They come in clusters. Not enough to trouble me."— Age forty-nine.

"When I was about forty-seven my menstrual cycles became very irregular and heavy. That's when the hot flashes started. At first I thought, 'Gee, they're not so bad.' But they got worse after my periods stopped. They start at my feet and work their way up. My blood feels like it's rushing to my head and then it recedes, leaving me weak and tired and cold. I also get dizzy. Never to the point where I pass out, just woozy. I work in a laundry and it can get uncomfortably steamy. When I have a flash at work I simply have to run out of there and take a deep *breath of fresh air. I used to get night sweats really bad. Not every night—just a few times a week. I'd wake up dripping wet. Lately I haven't been getting them at night. But I still get them intensely three or four times during the day."—Age fifty-two.*

"I began to have hot flashes after my total hysterectomy. They are really mean. The heat shoots up and you feel so hot. It's so intense. You feel like rolling in the snow."—Age forty-three.

"They started when I was forty-eight, after my periods stopped. At the beginning they were very intense. Sweat poured down my forehead and face. I couldn't stand being in crowds, especially on the packed subway going to work in summer. The feeling of being closed in and of other bodies crushed against me set them off. The sensations made me nervous. Several times I had to get out of the subway train and sit on the platform until a less crowded train came along. I had the sweats at night too. I'm a really sound sleeper though, and they never bothered me much. I still get the flashes about once a month— I think at about the time I would have ovulated if I were still menstruating. They can be set off anytime I'm feeling very warm or closed in."—Age sixty-four.

"My face gets beet red down to my chin and neck. I can consciously will myself to have a hot flash just by concentrating on it. I don't find it to be any big deal."—Age forty-nine.

"I had a hysterectomy at age thirty, but my ovaries were left intact. Without periods I had no idea whether or not I was nearing menopause. A little over two years ago I started having hot flashes. It's an overwhelming rise of heat. As it reaches its peak—in one to two minutes—I perspire very heavily on my face, head and the back of my neck. Then I feel clammy and chilled. My husband and I notice it most when I'm driving in the car, because I can't get out to cool off. He's really helpful and concerned. When I'm at the wheel and he sees me having one he helps me off with my coat and sweater. At night I

sometimes wake up wet—especially the back of my neck. Some flashes are more intense than others. I perspire more. Occasionally after a flash I feel washed out."—Age fifty-five.

"My flashes started after my period stopped. During the two years I had them I just continued going and doing. There was no change in my personality or in my outside social activities. We had a terraced apartment then. The flashes would hit suddenly and I'd be sopping wet, especially my head. So I'd step out on the terrace to cool off. Then I'd dry off just as fast. I never caught colds. Not even in the middle of the winter."— Age sixty-three.

Physical Changes During a Hot Flash

In medical terms hot flashes are known as a condition of vasomotor instability. This means that the diameters of the tiny blood vessels beneath your skin are widening and narrowing in an unpredictable fashion. When they dilate, blood rushes into them and the skin becomes warm and flushed; when they constrict, they leave a woman feeling cold and shivery. These abrupt vasomotor shifts affect the flow of blood and may be the cause of cold hands and feet, numbness and tingling, and possibly headaches and palpitations.[10,11]

Although flashes have been commonly observed in menopausal women for years, it was not until 1975 that a scientist, George Molnar, tried to document the actual physical changes that go on during a flashing episode. Molnar used his fifty-nine-year-old wife as a subject. He placed her on a nylon mesh bed mounted on an underbed scale (to measure water loss); and he kept careful records of her external skin temperature and internal body temperature, as well as her heart rate and the rate of perspiration. After observing his wife on four separate occasions, for a total of eight hot flashes, he made the following observations: 1. At the start of each flash his subject's heartbeat speeded up rapidly, but then slowed to normal by the time the flash ended. 2. There was a rise in skin temperature in her fingers, toes and cheeks. 3. Perspiration formed on the subject's forehead, nose and chest area (but little or none formed on her cheeks and legs). 4.

The internal body temperature remained normal, or dipped even slightly lower than usual. 5. The actual amount of sweat loss was quite small.[12]

Since Molnar's study, other scientists have conducted comparable experiments on women having hot flashes with similar results.

Trying to Find the Cause

Imagine that someone is tampering with your internal thermostat, setting it at a lower temperature. To reach this new, lower set point your body goes into action. Blood rushes into your blood vessels and causes the skin to heat up and perspire. As the perspiration evaporates, it cools you off and lowers your body temperature. This is what happens during a hot flash.

Why does this chain of events occur? No one knows for sure. Says Ann Voda, a nursing professor who has done a great deal of research on hot flashes: "If our prevalence figures have any credibility at all, the hot flash may have a positive biological value for women. Right now we don't know what that value is. Wouldn't it be wonderful if someday when the biological significance of the hot flash is appreciated, that women will welcome their first hot flash rather than adapt the negative present feelings associated with the hot flash?"[13]

While the exact cause of hot flashes is unclear, scientists are sure that they involve the hypothalamus—the brain's heat regulatory center—and that they are set off by declining estrogen levels.

The Estrogen Withdrawal Theory

Throughout your reproductive life high levels of estrogen flood into your system. Your body becomes "addicted" to this hormone. When the estrogen levels fall, as they do at menopause, you may experience withdrawal in the form of hot flashes. You might say that every woman is an estrogen "junky."

Adolescent girls with low levels of estrogen do not get hot flashes. Nor do women with congenitally low estrogen levels.[14] That's because it's necessary for estrogen levels to drop from high to low before hot flashes will occur. Flashes have been medically induced in both men and women when estrogen therapy is administered to them and then abruptly discontinued.[15]

According to the estrogen withdrawal theory, the more gradual the hormonal decline, the less severe the flashes. This seems to hold true. Those with surgical menopause, who have a sudden and dramatic plunge in estrogen levels, are most likely to experience severe hot flashes.[16] Heavier women, who produce more estrogen in their fat cells after menopause, tend to have an easier time with flashes than thinner women.[17]

The Role of LH, FSH and Other Hormones

The pituitary hormones FSH and LH rise dramatically in menopausal women. (For a full discussion of these hormones see Chapter 2.) So scientists at first surmised that these two hormones were somehow responsible for triggering hot flashes. No differences in FSH and LH levels could be found between women who had hot flashes and those who didn't. And this theory has since fallen by the wayside.[18,19,20,21]

In 1979 several researchers discovered that each time a woman has a flash her blood levels of LH (but not FSH) rise. Women would sometimes have a rise in LH levels without having a flash, but never vice versa. So LH didn't seem to cause the flashes—it just accompanied them.[22]

Scientists now suspect that an LH releasing factor originating from the hypothalamus may play a major role in setting off hot flashes. Several other hormones that influence the nervous and vascular systems are also under investigation.[23,24]

For now there are still many missing pieces in the hot flash puzzle. What scientists do know is that estrogen withdrawal seems to influence the hypothalamus so that the body's temperature set point is lowered and a flash occurs. As more and more pieces of the puzzle begin to fit together, scientists may be able to come up with newer and better treatments for women with severe flashes.

How Women Cope

How you cope with flashes depends a lot upon how severe they are. Much of the medical literature on the subject is based upon experiences of women who have had severe, life-disrupting problems. Luckily, the great majority of women have mild or only moderately uncomfortable hot flashes. They cope without doing anything special, or by making small adjustments in their daily routines.

Clothing

Something as simple as a change in wardrobe habits can make a big difference in your daily comfort. Avoid wearing synthetic fabrics such as polyesters and nylon, which trap perspiration. Cottons feel cooler to the touch and allow your skin to breathe.

Learn to dress in layers. That way you can remove and add clothing as you alternately perspire and cool off. A sleeveless or short-sleeved cotton blouse topped by a sweater or blazer is perfect in cooler weather.

You may have to temporarily shelve your favorite high necked dresses and turtleneck sweaters. Anything worn close to your neck may give you a trapped feeling when you're having a flash. V-necks and collars that can be unbuttoned at the throat are a wiser choice.

While you are at home, you may strip down and get as comfortable as you please. Confides one woman: "Sometimes I wear a bathing suit around the house—even in the middle of the winter!"

Bedclothes and linens should also be chosen with an eye toward comfort. Choose cool cottons for sheets, pillowcases and sleep wear. Some women feel most comfortable sleeping without any clothes, between cotton sheets.

"I've learned a little trick about night sweats," says one woman. "If I wear a very thin nighty and keep my feet outside of the covers when I'm falling asleep I am rarely awakened by them." Says another: "I always keep an extra nightgown on the table next to my bed. Then I don't have to get up out of bed to change in the middle of the night. I just reach out, grab for the extra nightgown, and roll over and go back to sleep. I rinse the damp one out in the morning." If your hot and cold spells are disturbing your partner's sleep, you might want to invest in an electric blanket with dual controls.

Body Coolers

An ice cold drink can help to cool you down during a hot flash. Keep a pitcher or thermos of ice water handy, whether it's on your desk at work or on your bedside table at home.

In Molnar's study his subject felt prompt relief when she cooled her cheeks off. You might try doing the same. Stand over a basin and splash cool water on your face or dip a compress into cold water and apply. You might want to keep a couple of picnic freezer packs handy in your home freezer (they contain a cooling agent and are usually used to keep insulated picnic bags cool). These may be wrapped in a washcloth and placed against your cheeks whenever necessary.

One woman came up with an ingenious cooling method of her own: "I use one of the masks they sell for sinus headaches you can boil them in water to retain heat or put them in the freezer to retain cold. I keep mine in the freezer. When I'm having a flash I come downstairs and grab it out of the fridge and then lie down with it on my face. It's tremendously cooling to my face—which is the hottest part of me."

Another woman keeps a cold, wet washcloth in a plastic container near her bedside: "I apply the cloth to my forehead and cheeks when I am wakened by a hot flash in the middle of the night."

The feeling of cool, moving air on your skin, as from an air conditioner or electric fan, can also bring relief. One obvious and simple solution is to carry a fan in your purse. Miniature battery-run fans are also convenient to use at work or when you travel.

If you're lucky enough to be lounging near a pool or on the beach you can always take a quick dip. At home a cool shower will accomplish the same thing.

Mental Imagery

In one study of hot flashes one of the subjects said that she found it helpful to "tell her flashes to go away." Another said that she used visual imagery, imagining how it would feel to sit in a snow bank.[25] Perhaps you can close your eyes and imagine yourself wandering through a swirling snowstorm, or dunking into a clear, icy lake.

Above all, try to remain calm. Getting excited over the fact that you are having a flash may only aggravate the situation, and may even make the flash last longer.[26] Instead, kick off your shoes, loosen or remove your clothing, and breathe in and out deeply and rhythmically. Remind yourself that this flash can't really hurt you in any way and that it will soon be over.

Feelings of Embarrassment

Some women are self-conscious about having hot flashes in public situations. They feel as if everyone is watching them. If you are wondering whether your hot flashes are obvious to others, just look in the mirror as you're having one. While flashes are sometimes physically apparent, they often do not look as bad as they feel.

Try not to be embarrassed about flashes. They are a normal, natural part of growing older, and they happen to almost every woman. Admitting to people matter-of-factly that you are having a hot flash is probably the best way to deal with it. Says one saleswoman who deals with the public all day long: "When I'm waiting on a customer, I'll say, 'Whoops, I'm having a hot flash'—and we'll usually joke and make light of the whole thing." Says another, who works as an office secretary: "When I'm having a hot flash at work and my temperature rises, it steams my eyeglasses. My co-workers know what's going on because I remove my sweater and keep wiping my glasses to get the fog off of them. They sometimes tease me. But I don't get offended. It's a gentle teasing, a way of reaching out and acknowledging what I'm going through."

Of course, it's not always easy to shrug off a flash with great aplomb. Unexpected bouts of flushing and perspiration are difficult for anyone to deal with, and may be especially so for the woman who is a fastidious type and who likes her life to be neat and orderly. The professional who must face the public daily may feel very differently about her hot flashes than the woman who works at home. "My kids comment aloud each and every time I have a hot flash," says one kindergarten teacher, who has learned to take it all in good humor. "They keep asking me why my face gets so red. So I tell them that I'm just feeling very warm."

Some women choose to minimize the whole experience: "If you perspire, wipe it. If you have to change your nighty, change it. Don't make a big deal of it." Others ignore it: "I just accepted it and waited for it to be over." Still others find that talking about it and sharing their concerns with others make them feel a lot less alone and frightened: "If menopause makes you feel strange and unique and you shrink away from others you'll have a hard time. I find that sharing it makes it a lot easier." Don't be surprised if other women are as eager as you to discuss this little-mentioned part of their lives. You may even want to join a menopause support group or form one on your own (for advice on how, see page 87).

In one Welsh mining village, women see flashes as a sign of good health and may tend to brag about and exaggerate them.[27] Few women in this country feel overjoyed at the prospect of having hot flashes. But for some, they are a source of pride. Says one fifty-two-year-old. "I say it's a badge of honor, to have gone through so much and reached this point of life. Someone terribly shy or conscious of how other people feel about them will have more trouble with hot flashes. As for me, I say, take me for what I am—or leave me."

Medical Remedies

Estrogen

Women who have severe, life-disrupting hot flashes may want to consider estrogen replacement therapy. Estrogen is currently the only drug medically known to put an end to hot flashes. It is, in fact, nearly 100 percent effective.[28,29] Estrogen replacement therapy remains a controversial method because of its association with increased incidences of cancer. The hormone is usually given in the smallest doses for the shortest possible time. An in-depth look at the pros and cons of estrogen therapy is presented in Chapter 6.

Clonidine

Some women cannot tolerate estrogen, or can't take it because of their health or family history. In such cases a doctor may prescribe clonidine. This drug is used to treat high blood pressure, but it also appears to control hot flashes. It is an especially good choice for hypertensive women who are also troubled by severe hot flashes. Clonidine may have some unpleasant side effects, however. In one study of ten menopausal women treated with clonidine for severe hot flashes, participants complained of such discomforts as dryness of the mouth, severe fatigue, headaches, irritability, dizziness and insomnia. Furthermore, clonidine was found to be only 46 percent effective in alleviating hot flashes.[30]

Progestin

Progestin is a synthetic form of the female hormone progesterone. It is a more effective alternative to estrogen than clonidine. Studies have found that progestin brings total or significant relief in about 90 percent of women treated. It may, however, cause a woman to experience irregular spotting.[31,32] The current trend is to administer estrogen and progestin in a cyclical fashion, much as they are released during the menstrual cycle. But progestin alone may be effective for women who cannot be treated with estrogen.

Sedatives and Tranquilizers

Sedatives and tranquilizers are also prescribed as an alternative to estrogen. They may relax and calm the nerves, and may help a woman to get some much-needed sleep. While they can be helpful, they are also potentially addictive. And they dull everyday life experiences along with the flashes.

Sometimes women are given combination drugs that include sedatives or tranquilizers and antispasmodics (to relax muscles). Bellergal is the name of one commonly administered combination tablet.[33,34]

Sedatives and tranquilizers may alleviate hot flashes by blurring a woman's senses. But they don't actually eliminate the symptoms. Exercise, yoga and stress reduction techniques, which are described elsewhere in this book, may also help a woman to relax.

Nonmedical Alternatives

Herbal Remedies

Natural herbs have been used over the centuries to treat all sorts of ailments. In fact, many of today's synthetically manufactured drugs were originally created by mimicking the properties of herbs. Holistic doctors, naturopaths, herbalists and other alternative healers still use herbs for medicinal purposes, including the alleviation of menopausal hot flashes.

Herbs can be potent, and some may even be toxic, advises one naturopath who practices in upstate New York. "Two or three cups of herbal tea a day aren't likely to hurt you, but if you wish to experiment with various herbs you should do so only under the supervision of an experienced physician or herbalist."

Herbs which have been reported helpful in dealing with menopause include: sarsaparilla, licorice, red raspberry, cramp bark, black cohosh, damiana, don quai, ginseng, squaw vine and false unicorn root.[35,36,37,38,39] These herbs are said to contain estrogen as well as to stimulate the body to produce its own female hormones. They are sold in health food stores in dried or powdered form, and may be made into teas or capsules. Herbalists usually recommend a combination of several of these ingredients. Some stores sell prepackaged blends of herbs tailored specifically for menopausal symptoms.

Vitamin Therapy

Several vitamins have been reported by women to help relieve hot flashes. These include vitamins E, B, C and bioflavonoids. They are usually taken together in supplements and proponents say it may take several weeks before a woman will see results.[40,41] As with herbs, vitamins in large doses are potentially toxic, and should be taken only under the guidance of a knowledgable health care provider.

Vitamin E is by far the most widely touted of the vitamin remedies. While promising studies were done on this vitamin in the 1940s and early 1950s, they are outdated in terms of current knowledge about hot flashes and their research methods. The only information available today is based on testimonials from women who claim that vitamin E has helped to ease or eliminate their hot flashes.[42]

Vitamin E cannot be taken by everyone. Large supplements may be dangerous for those with high blood pressure, diabetes or rheumatic heart conditions. It can cause side effects including gastric upset, blurred vision, blood clots, high blood pressure and breast development in men and women.[43,44]

Natural sources of vitamin E include whole grain breads and cereals; wheat germ; corn, soybean, safflower and wheat germ oils; beans; peas; dark green, leafy vegetables; and eggs.

Vitamin B complex and vitamin C are together described as a stress formula.[45] Vitamin B complex is actually fifteen vitamins which are grouped together because they appear in most of the same foods. Brewer's yeast is an excellent source of B vitamins, as are whole grain breads and cereals and wheat germ. B vitamins are also present in milk, meat, poultry, green leafy vegetables, beans and peas.

Sources of vitamin C include citrus fruits, bell peppers, tomatoes, honeydew melon, cantaloupe, rose hips, broccoli, cauliflower, cabbage and strawberries. Bioflavonoids (said to enhance the effects of vitamin C) are contained in the white inner skin of citrus fruits.

Most vitamin proponents recommend a daily calcium supplement both for its bone-building properties and for its ability to help relieve tension. A full discussion of the benefits of calcium during menopause will be presented in Chapter 7.

A Self-Limiting Symptom

Whether or not herbs and vitamins actually work to reduce hot flashes remains to be proven. Some physicians feel that their effectiveness is largely due to a placebo effect. That is, the woman believes they will work—and so they do. "You can't knock these other things proposed," says one gynecologist. "A placebo can change reception in the brain."

The fact is, hot flashes clear up all by themselves no matter what steps a woman does—or does not—take. In most cases they are at their worst for a year or two and then either disappear or slowly phase themselves out. Within five years the majority of women are completely finished with hot flashes, and those who have them longer find them to be mild and very infrequent.

Remarks one sixty-four-year-old veteran of the hot flashes: "If I didn't know that a flash was normal, all of that flushing and sweating would have made me petrified. But I knew what the cause was, and that they wouldn't last forever. My advice to other women who are going through menopause is this: don't be alarmed by flashes. Bear with them and try to be as calm as possible. It's nothing really serious. Nothing bad will happen to you."

Chapter 4

The
Middle-Age
Blues

"The stages of life in this country are not exactly well-defined. We generally grow from being too-young to still-young to looking-younger-than-our age. We do not greet middle age; we admit to it."—Ellen Goodman, syndicated columnist.[1]

Mental illness is no more prevalent during menopause than at any other stage of life. If you are a reasonably well-adjusted person you are not likely to develop severe emotional problems now.

Some women do say that they experience a temporary emotional slump during these transitional years. They may feel blue and moody, and lack their former "oomph." "Some days I'm soaring in high spirits and others I feel down in the dumps," says one forty-nine-year-old. "I feel more stressed, more sensitive, more easily triggered to anger and tears. Little things or remarks may set me off, although I know rationally that I'm over reacting. I have trouble falling asleep, which I never have before. Sometimes I feel paranoid. I tire easily. I feel fragile, like I'm going to fall apart."

Not everyone has these out-of-sync feelings, but they're common enough among menopausal women to have become a subject of medical investigation. In fact, scientists have observed that the following physical and emotional symptoms often occur together in clusters: mood swings, insomnia, depression, irritability, fatigue, dizziness, headaches, palpitations, and numbness or tingling in the extremities. Some have even labeled this a menopause "syndrome."

Are these symptoms triggered by declining hormone levels? If they are, hormone therapy should effectively put an end to them. Are they a reaction to the emotional stresses of the middle years? In that case counseling or antidepressants should help. Or are they simply the result of aging, and not related to menopause at all?

Scientists can't seem to agree on any one answer. In some studies estrogen has helped to clear up emotional symptoms and to restore the subjects' feelings of well-being; but in others a placebo plus counseling and support were equally—if not more—effective than hormone replacement therapy.[2] To add to the confusion, one questionnaire survey found that men and women of similar ages both suffer from minor complaints usually blamed on menopause.[3,4]

Chances are that there's some truth to all of these explanations. The mind and body can exert a powerful influence on each other. And the so-called menopause syndrome may be the combined result of a number of causes—physical, emotional and cultural.

If you suffer from a number of the aforementioned complaints you should, of course, consult with your physician. A thorough medical examination can rule out conditions—such as thyroid or blood sugar imbalances—which may cause similar symptoms.

Physical Factors/Can Hormones Affect Your Moods?

What woman hasn't felt inordinately touchy and then checked her calendar to find that, "Oh, yes, it's that time of the month"? Minor mood swings coincide with the female ebb and flow of hormones. You may feel most energetic and creative before ovulation, when estrogen levels are high, and more lethargic and blue premenstrually, when hormone levels drop. It is not surprising that mood swings occur at menopause, when hormones are in a similar state of flux.

According to one expert in the field of PMS (premenstrual syndrome) there is a subgroup of women—about 10 percent of the female population—who are exquisitely sensitive to hormone changes. They show serious signs of depression both premenstrually and in the period immediately following childbirth. This same subgroup is also likely to experience severe depression at menopause, when their estrogen levels again take a dip.[5]

As they approach menopause many women complain of exaggerated premenstrual symptoms. Mood swings, bloating and breast tenderness may be more pronounced than usual. "A few days before my period arrives I may burst into tears if you just look at me the wrong way," says one forty-three-year-old. "I snap at my family for little things. The bloating definitely contributes to my increased nervousness. I feel myself physically expanding, as if I am going to explode. The retained fluid also gives me headaches. When I begin to menstruate, all of this tension is released."

As we've already noted, many emotional symptoms actually stem from severe hot flashes and night sweats. A woman whose sleep is repeatedly interrupted is likely to experience insomnia and to feel cranky, tired and depressed during the day. The dilation and contraction of her blood vessels during each flash may contribute to headaches, palpitations, and sensations of tingling or numbness in her extremities. Estrogen is often successful in lifting women's spirits because of its domino effect. By ending hot flashes it enables a woman to get a good night's sleep. That means that she will feel happier and more refreshed the next day.

Emotional Factors/Women at Life's Crossroads

It's easy to blame your shifting hormones for all that ails you. Menopause comes at a difficult juncture in most women's lives. It is a time of transition and change. These changes can generate a lot of stress. And stress can cause the exact same constellation of physical and emotional symptoms that have been attributed to menopause.

Many people in their forties and fifties pause to take inventory of their past attainments and ask themselves some weighty questions: "Who am I?" "What have I accomplished in my life?" "Where am I going from here?" Like adolescence, middle age can be an emotional mine field. Most get through the passage unscathed. But they may find that unresolved problems from the past are churned up along the way.

In the midst of this, women must come face to face with the physical changes of menopause. Most women are happy to part with menstruation and childbearing. But the loss of periods is a concrete reminder of aging. The childbearing era is over. There is no turning back the clock. Thoughts about aging and death may be more difficult to sweep under the rug.

"I think a lot more about my mortality lately. When you are young you think you will live forever. I really don't have periods of dwelling to excess. But I've started to think about my life—where am I going and where have I gotten. I thought, 'Hey, more than half of my life is over!' All of these thoughts keep seeping through the cracks of everyday life."

"You start noticing changes in your body—gaining weight, periods getting shorter and less frequent. People start calling you 'ma'am.' The kids at college look through you, unless you're a professor. You say to yourself: 'Oh my god, it's really happening.'"

The loss of monthly cycles represents the end of an important part of your female identity. And it's natural to be disturbed about that:

"The choice of having any more children is no longer mine to make, though for all intents and purposes it was all over for me long ago by choice. It's like being a child with two fistfuls of cookies and a full belly. Yet she still eyes the chocolate cupcake in the bakery window."

Your reaction to your last menstrual period will probably be influenced by your childbearing history. If you've had as many children as you wanted and enjoyed raising them to maturity, you'll likely be ready to close the chapter on mothering. Those with PMS, heavy and painful periods, or fibroids and endometriosis (conditions which clear up following menopause) may greet menopause with genuine relief. Women who have undergone tubal ligations have already wrestled with the fertility issue, and are less likely to feel emotional about the loss of periods.

One mother of six, plagued by the fear of another pregnancy, says that she welcomed her menopause: "For the first time I could truly enjoy making love to my husband." But another, who was never able to conceive, felt this way:

"It makes me sad. I have never borne a child. But it's always been in the back of my mind that one day I might. Even that hope—slim as it might be—is over. A fantasy never to be realized. This was followed by a period of acceptance. Not in a negative sense. Menopause is a fact of life. And life goes on."

Menopause tolls the final chime on the reproductive clock. And those who have postponed childbearing may be distressed to find that time has made their ultimate decision for them. Even the woman who deliberately chose not to have children may find herself reassessing her life's decision: "I'm not sorry. I see my friends suffering with their teenagers while we've gone off to the Riviera and taken up waterskiing. But yes, it did make me reflect on the whole baby issue again."

The Empty-Nest Syndrome

During your menopausal years your full-grown children may be setting out on their own paths. When a woman has spent so many years nurturing others, this stage can come as quite a jolt.

"My daughter and I fought like cats and dogs. We never seemed to see eye-to-eye on anything. But after she got married

and moved out I went into a very bad depression. Suddenly the house seemed so quiet and empty without her. I cried for two weeks straight."

Full-time homemakers with few interests outside of their families may be hardest hit by the empty nest syndrome.[6] They may at first feel disoriented and unneeded. "It's like being on an open highway without any signposts," says one woman who stayed home for twenty years to rear her youngsters. "If you don't know where you're going it can be very depressing."

All of the time spent chauffeuring, cooking and caring for youngsters is past. Where once you had to juggle your schedule to find a free hour, you may now seem to have too much time on your hands. Some women have to consciously learn how to relax and enjoy this bonanza of free time in a constructive way.

With the influence of the women's movement, mothers today are more conscious about the need to maintain an identity outside of their families. More and more are returning to work or school while their children are still quite young. But careers and outside interests do not grant full immunity to the empty nest syndrome. Even this busy career woman feels a keen sense of loss as her children begin to take flight:

"In the course of raising three children, I've only taken off a total of four years from work. But my identification with my children is strong. I feel a need to hold them close to me, not out of desperation, but because I love mothering so much. Lately I have powerful fears that something bad will happen to them. My oldest is away at college and will not be moving back home. My sixteen-year-old began driving this year and I'm terrified that she will be in a car crash. My thirteen-year-old rides her bike further from home, and I'm afraid for her safety. I think my fears are related to the end of their childhood. I'm not sure how to react to their new independence. When I work out my relationship with my oldest child it will probably come more easily with the others."

As many a middle-aged woman can tell you, the empty nest often turns out to be a blessing in disguise. Now is the time to do all of those things you've always wanted to do, but said you never had the time for. For some this means traveling, hobbies or civic activities. Others plunge back into school or work, earning new degrees and forging ahead in brand-new careers. The working mother who was always torn between the needs of her family and her job may find that life is less of a balancing act now that the kids are grown.

"At first I was sad about this phase of my life. But then I began to look at it in a positive way. It's an interesting time. I never dwelt as much on just me before. I guess you can call this chapter of my life, 'Mom finally does her own thing.'"

"When Laura moves out I'm converting her bedroom to an office. At last I'll be able to move my books and papers off the dining room table and get cracking on my Ph.D. dissertation."

"It's great having the kids on their own. I can come and go as I please. I like having them visit and helping out with the grandchildren. But I love my privacy and my free and easy schedule."

Not all children at home are old enough for independence. Some middle-aged mothers bemoan what it's like to cope with teenage children who are going through an identity crisis of their own.

"The stress of having teenagers is getting to me. You want to protect them from making big mistakes, but they think they know it all. My daughter is into drugs and thinks our values are antiquated. I can't kick her out—that would be like throwing her to the wolves. But I can't condone her friends or lifestyle either. Between worrying about them and what I want to do with the rest of my life I haven't been sleeping or eating. It

takes a tremendous emotional toll. I feel like I'm close to having a mental breakdown."

"My sixteen-year-old doesn't seem to take anything in life seriously. His grades in school are slipping and he's hanging around with a wild crowd. He recently announced to us that he wasn't going to college. He wants to be a rock musician. I wouldn't mind that so much, but he doesn't even study his music seriously. Do you think that nature invented teenagers so that we wouldn't mind letting go of them when the time comes?"

Grown children may add to mid-life stresses in other ways. You may not like their choice of mates for example, or their decision to live with one another, or to marry at a young age. The values your children adopt may be diametrically opposed to the ones you sought to impart. One woman was heartbroken when her daughter, a college graduate, joined an Eastern religious sect and took a vow of celibacy. "We had always taught her to question everyone and everything, that teachers and authority figures were not always right. And now she's joined a herd of followers."

Some adult children don't ever seem to want to leave the comfort of their parents' nest. They may come and go at will (often with grandchildren in tow), interrupting their parents' schedules and privacy. "The only thing worse than having your children move out is having them move back in again," one woman says half-jokingly.

Children may thrust you into the role of mother-in-law or grandmother. And these new roles can bring added stresses as well as joys. Quips one sprightly forty-eight-year-old: "No one asked me if I was ready to become a grandma. They just went ahead and made me one."

A Role Reversal with Aging Parents

As your parents age your relationship with them may become reversed. If they are elderly and infirm, you may now have to become the nurturer, providing for their physical and financial needs. This can be an enormous source of emotional and economic strain. And the middle-aged daughter may feel torn between obligations to herself, her family and her elderly parents.

"I took one year off from work. I spent the year alone crying, writing in my journal and reading. I didn't know what I was going to do or where I was going to be. Issues with my mom had to be sorted out. She is seventy-five and depends upon me for many things. She will be dying soon. She has cancer and Parkinson's disease. My oldest daughter is a senior in college. I have to work it through—this letting go of her. My husband is also evaluating his life and his work. I feel squeezed between the generations. I feel responsible for my mother, my children, everyone. All of these pressures hit me at once."

"At ninety-one my mother's health is deteriorating. She lives by herself in an apartment and has always been very proud of her independence. I visit her every day, and she's so appreciative. It's always been hard for her to express emotions. But for the first time in years she told me how much she loves me. Lately she's not eating as much, and is getting terribly thin. I think to myself, 'Maybe she'll get her appetite back.' But it's not a realistic expectation. Whether or not to put her into a nursing home is a very difficult decision. She's at the point where she can no longer take care of herself. She needs constant care. Sometimes I can't sleep thinking about my mom and her changing condition. I just don't know what to do. My mom is so dependent on me."

The death of one's parents is a traumatic event. As a child they were your protectors, an invincible shield against mortality. Now it's your turn to move to the helm of three generations: an honor of dubious distinction. "In your teens, twenties and thirties you think you're never going to die," comments one fifty-year-old. "The generations ahead of you were life's buffers. Facing death is a hard thing to do. But it shapes your life. You think about what has to get done."

Marriage and Mid-Life Crisis

Marital satisfaction is said to be highest before the birth of children and again after the last offspring walks out the door.[7] The empty nest often converts to a comfortable love nest, feathered with travel, social engagements and lazy Sunday mornings in bed. Many couples describe a period of renewed intimacy, much like a second honeymoon.

"My husband and I are very close. We share moods—we think like one. Our son is on his own and doing well and our daughter is well on her way to independence. Now we're thinking in terms of what we want to do with the rest of our lives. It's an exciting passage for us. It's a good time."

A husband can buoy up his wife during her sometimes stormy middle years. A good marriage is an important source of love and emotional support. Women with secure relationships seem to have fewer problems with menopause.

Your husband's attitude toward menopause may be influenced by how sensitive his own father was to his wife's menopause. Men, too, have to be educated on the physical and emotional changes that occur at this time. They have also been influenced by myths, stereotypes and misinformation. Perhaps you can share what you are reading or learning on the subject with your husband. Never having experienced menstrual cycles or hormonal upheavals himself, menopause may be difficult for him to understand. An open line of communication between you is very important now.

But sometimes a man is floundering in a full-blown middle-age crisis of his own. Your husband, too, may be distressed at physical signs of aging. And he may feel an urgency about getting things accomplished in his life before it is too late. The stresses in his life may translate into feelings of depression, fatigue, irritability and sleeplessness.

Most middle-aged men take a hard look at their lives in terms of career goals. If a man hasn't "made it" by this time he may feel like a failure. He may bury himself totally in his work in a last-ditch effort to make it to the top. Even those who reach the pinnacle of their careers can feel despondent.

The rewards for a lifetime of effort may seem empty, and the highly successful businessman may ask himself: "Is that all there is?"

The middle-aged man may see younger and less experienced workers leapfrog over him for prized promotions. Stuck in an unrewarding, dead-end job, he may feel powerless to leave it. There are valued pensions and health benefits to consider. And besides, who would hire a man at his age? Of course, the same stresses apply to career women in their middle years. And many share the same frustrations as their male counterparts.

Says one woman, whose husband is acting irritable and having trouble sleeping: "He won't admit it, but he seems to be going through some mid-life emotional changes. I'm sure a lot of it has to do with his job. He really hates it. But at this stage of the game where can he go? He's in a real bind. We bicker with each other all of the time. It's like we're in a contest of wills. He wants to be the decision-maker at home. But I'm feeling pretty assertive and strong-willed myself lately."

Men and women appear to move in opposite, but complementary directions at mid-life. A man tends to become more nurturing, permitting his softer side to show, while a woman is apt to grow more assertive and self-assured. Sometimes the mid-life goals of men and women are at direct odds. He may feel "burnt out" after working a lifetime. She may feel liberated from the time-consuming needs of home and children. While his dream is to retire early and take off to a retirement community in Florida, hers is to charge into the hustle and bustle of the work world.

Often spouses blame each other for their own shortcomings and disappointments. They may try to prove their own worth and attractiveness by seeking out other partners. Extramarital affairs and divorce rates are particularly high at this time of life.[8] And the story of the staid corporate executive who trades in wife, job and security to start a brand-new life with a younger woman is all too familiar. Some couples find that they have little left in common after their children move out, and so choose this time to separate.

For some women there is the ultimate separation—widowhood. The loss of a beloved spouse usually comes as a devastating shock. Says one recent widow: "When you divorce, you probably have some say in the matter, but for me there was no choice at all. It just happened with a bang."

Divorce and Widowhood

The woman who is divorced or widowed after twenty or thirty years of marriage may feel as if the rug has been pulled out from under her. She may feel lonely and isolated in a world filled with couples—a fifth wheel among former married friends. Scoffs one recent widow: "Your old married friends call to ask you out for lunch dates, but never for dinner." Financial questions and major decisions may seem overwhelming when you are not used to facing them alone. Full-time homemakers may be forced out into the workplace with few skills and even less self-confidence. In dealing with these hardships many women say that they discover an inner strength that surprises them.

"A couple of years ago I got divorced. I had spent most of my married life as a full-time housewife raising our five children. Now I didn't want to stay home any more. There was no husband coming home to me at night. I needed a new point of focus. At first I worked for a few hours a week. I found that all of my working skills came back to me beautifully. Then I worked full-time. I went back to school at night to get training as an interior decorator and I am really enjoying it. It was a lot more difficult to get it together on my own. It's scary and exciting. I've found that I've grown a lot and have really enjoyed the challenge."

"The loss of my husband was a tremendous letdown. I didn't know which way to turn. My oldest daughter was a newlywed, and she made it clear that I couldn't move in with them. My son just got out of the army, and he told me that he would only live with me for a few months before moving out on his own. My married friends called a lot at first, and invited me places. But then the invitations came less and less frequently. I felt stranded. I wasn't needed by anyone any more. I had to *start all over. I had to pick up all of the pieces myself. No one was going to do it for me.*

"After about two years of being depressed I pulled myself together. I gave myself a good cry and then said, 'that's enough.' I joined singles organizations, took trips and went on cruises. Not with the idea of getting a mate—just to keep busy. Within a year I met a man and we got married. You can't replace your old mate. It's a completely new phase. But in some respects my second marriage is better than the first.

"In retrospect I'm glad my children made me rely on myself rather than on them. If I leaned on them, I never would have made the effort to create a life of my own."

"My husband died seven years ago, when I was fifty-one. I relocated to live near my son and daughter-in-law. I found I couldn't depend on them. I didn't get along with my daughter-in-law as much as I had hoped. She wouldn't let my grandchild come over as often as I would have liked. She resents my intrusion. So I decided I had to have a life of my own. I needed less time to dwell upon myself and my losses. I got myself a job at a day-care center. I also do volunteer work for handicapped children and am active in a community arts committee. There are so many people out there in need and there's so much you can give. When you're widowed you have to get out there and meet people and do things. Don't watch TV and cry behind closed doors. Call a friend, have people over for dinner, go out and volunteer or get a job. Everyone walks around with a pocketful of troubles. Nobody wants to sit around listening to yours."

Our Youth-Worshipping Culture

Menopause itself is only one possible source of mid-life stress. Grown children, aging parents, marital discord, divorce and widowhood can all contribute to feelings of anxiety. Added to these is society's dim view of the aging female.

Our culture places a premium on youth. Flawless young faces grace the pages of fashion magazines, while middle-aged women are depicted as victims of arthritis, hemorrhoids or slipping dentures. "Look years younger" . . . "Hide wrinkles"

. . . "Cover gray" . . . exhort the TV jingles. We are a nation that spends more on cosmetics than on education.[9]

There is a strong double standard at play. Men in their fifties and sixties can still be the romantic heroes of film and stage. A little gray at the temples only serves to make them more dashing. And the middle-aged woman? She is usually portrayed as a nagging shrew or overbearing mother-in-law. Rarely do we see a vibrant, sexually attractive middle-aged female taking center stage.

These public images of middle-aged women affect the way women feel about themselves in private. The word "menopause" has come to have negative connotations: "We used to call my place of employment 'menopause manor,'" recalls one woman. "It was a derogatory term, referring to the fact that most of the employees were women in their fifties and upwards. Only now, in retrospect, do I realize how ageist that remark was." Says a forty-year-old: "I was recently at a heated business meeting when several of the female employees walked out. One of my male colleagues turned to me and said: 'Oh, you can't expect anything intelligent from those women. They're all going through the changes.' I felt irate. Is this how men view us as we grow older?"

Menopausal women may not be taken seriously enough—even in the physician's office. This was found to be true in a study of nine family physicians treating fifty-two middle-aged married couples. The couples complained of five medical problems (back pain, headaches, dizziness, chest pain and fatigue). The researchers reported that when the men complained of these ailments they received a more extensive physical workup than women.[10]

While declining estrogen levels at menopause are universal, the negative view of menopause and the aging female is not. Anthropologist Marsha Flint studied menopausal symptoms among 483 women of the Rajput caste in India. She chose the Rajputs, a well-nourished, healthy people, so that poor nutrition wouldn't skew her study results. Flint found that few of the women had any problems with menopause beyond their menstrual changes. Depression, dizziness or any of the other symptoms associated with menopause were not reported. In fact, most of these women looked forward eagerly to reaching menopause, or else were very positive about having attained it.

Why were the Rajputs so positive about menopause? Rajput women must live in "purda"—that is, they must wear veils and remain segregated from all men with the exception of their husbands. Only after menopause are they permitted to leave the women's quarters to publicly visit, drink brew and joke with the men in their society. While women in the U.S. are, in a sense, punished for reaching menopause, the Rajput women are rewarded for it. [11,12,13]

Other cultures similarly reward middle-aged females. Their wisdom and advice is often valued in an extended family. And they are often granted singular honors, such as the right to tread upon sacred ground, participate in important rituals, and to become tribal healers.

No one in the U.S. would want to live in "purda" or be restricted from community life during their childbearing years. On the other hand, our society has a long way to go in recognizing the values of maturity and age. Negative views of menopause may add to a woman's dread of this event and may even magnify the discomforts she experiences. In a comprehensive review on the subject one author asks this question: is it our society that has the neurotic symptoms rather than the menopausal woman? [14]

In the view of two psychologists, writing in the *Journal of the American Geriatrics Society*: "The self-image of the menopausal woman may be enhanced if she believes that menopause is an adaptive process, particularly responsible for her superior longevity, and is not a symptom of physiologic decline." [15]

Changes in the Wind

Over half of the people in the United States today are over the age of thirty. We are an aging population. And this trend is expected to accelerate over the next several decades.

The graying of America is bound to have a profound effect on society's attitudes toward aging. The baby boomers, who thumbed their noses at the older generation in the sixties, are now beginning to gray at the temples themselves. This segment of men and women, now in their thirties and forties, were notorious political activists. And they're bound to upset the applecart on aging issues as well. Their motto for the next decade may very well be: "Never trust anyone under forty."

In response to sheer numbers, magazines, clothing manufacturers and filmmakers will undoubtedly start aiming their goods and services toward a maturing population. Images of chic, middle-aged women are likely to flash across our TV screens and be sprinkled liberally through the fashion pages.

The women's movement is also maturing, and beginning to focus on issues beyond the childbearing years. More books and literature on middle-aged women are being published. And the subject of menopause is being discussed among women more openly than ever before. "My daughter won't have the same problems as I did," says one woman. "I didn't know anything. I talk to my three girls about what it's like to go through the changes. Sometimes we joke about it. It's all very casually treated. It's important that it not be such a big mystery to them."

Women in their forties and fifties today are just beginning to reap the benefits of these positive changes. They are learning that age can have no limits, and that the middle years can be an exciting block of time.

"Self-confidence can grow as you age. I began to feel my womanhood in my thirties. Life began in my forties. I had increased self-esteem and confidence. I went back to work at a job on a newspaper. I was no longer afraid to meet people. Before I felt scared and shy inside. I always smiled. No one could tell. But I know there's a difference inside—about the way I feel about myself. I have less concern about people and what they think. No one else can decide what's right for me."

"I don't feel my age. Fifty-five used to be old and gray. Women today are youthful. Their bodies are active. They have a better sense of what they want to do. I have more self-confidence. Not like I used to be."

"I wouldn't want to make all of life's choices over again. I wouldn't want to be a teenager or collegian or entering the job

*market today. I made my career choice. I'm happy and re-
spected by my colleagues and I still have retirement to look
forward to and lovely things to accomplish. I think it's a real
crisis when you feel as if you have nothing more to do in life,
that at fifty or sixty there are no goals. When I retire I am going
to organize a theatre group of handicapped children. We're
going to go into all of the schools and show people that handicapped children have the same feelings and joys as others. I
only hope that I have my health so that I can accomplish these
things."*

*"Age is only a number. My mother at fifty-one seemed an
old lady. I'm older than that and I look better than ever. My
granddaughter thinks I'm young—just like her daddy. Being
older can be a wonderful thing. Like a second honeymoon with
your husband. It's a time to travel and enjoy. Why mope about
it, for godsakes!"*

More women in conspicuous places are flaunting their
years and breaking down age barriers. They are writing best-
sellers, winning Oscars, entering marathons and running political races. When feminist Gloria Steinem turned forty, a
reporter told her that she didn't look her age. She replied to
this backhanded compliment with: "This is what forty looks
like. We've been lying so long, who would know." At fifty,
Steinem posed for *People* magazine in a bathtub full of bub-
bles and later threw an enormous birthday bash at New York's
Waldorf Astoria hotel. She flung this classic remark at re-
porters: "Fifty is what forty used to be."[16]

Older is definitely better according to author Gail Sheehy.
After interviewing hundreds of people across the country, she
found that mature people scored consistently higher in terms
of personal well-being. In her book, *Pathfinders,* she writes:
"Middle-aged men get to play and cry. Middle-aged women
get to tell their mothers off and leave notes for their husbands:
'Put in oven at 350° for 30 minutes—I'm off to the airport.'
It is, in fact, the middle-aged who have the tennis elbows and
the year-round tanning line from that fling in Jamaica or the

deck of their weekend place." And who are the people who go "off the charts in happiness"? They are the middle-aged women—"just past menopause; friends with, but unconfined by now-grown children; and feeling a firm sense of their own identity for the first time."[17]

Chapter 5
Getting
"Up" and
Out

The middle years can be a highly stressful time for women. There are so many new things happening to you at once—from changes within your body, to the loss of familiar social roles. If enough changes occur at one time, a woman can feel as if her circuits are overloaded. And she may begin to develop a spectrum of "nervous" symptoms (i.e., depression, irritability, insomnia, fatigue, dizziness, headaches and cold, numb or tingling extremities).

Of course, everyone feels stressed on occasion. Stress is a normal part of daily life. And it can be a positive and invigorating force. Stress gets your juices flowing so that you can solve a difficult problem, meet a deadline, or get an injured child quickly to the emergency room. It makes the actress shine on stage, and gives the track star a boost so that she can get a leg over the finish line.

Stress can be triggered by happy events, such as planning

a wedding or starting a new job. Or it can be triggered by sorrowful ones, like the death of a parent or spouse. No matter what the cause, stress results in the same physiologic responses: your muscles tighten, your heart speeds up, the rate of your breathing increases, and adrenaline pumps through your system. Your body is primed to go into action. Scientists call this the "fight-or-flight" response.

These physical reactions have helped the human species to survive down through the ages. In the beginning, this sudden surge of alertness and energy enabled the cave man to fight or flee from attacking predators at a moment's notice. While today you are not likely to fend a bear off at your doorstep, or to flee into the woods with a lion at your heels, what you may be wrestling with are emotional problems· Should you go back to work? Will you have to place your ailing parent in a nursing home? How do you deal with rebellious teenagers? With these types of stresses, there is no way to let off steam. Instead, your riled emotions may build to a point where you start feeling frayed around the edges.

A stressful situation can cause you to hyperventilate without being conscious of it. That is, you breathe too rapidly so that you are taking in too much oxygen and releasing too much carbon dioxide. The resulting imbalance can cause dizziness; numb, cold, or tingling extremities; and sometimes fainting. Tensed-up muscles in your neck and back may lead to headaches and backaches.

"I discovered a breast lump (which later turned out to be a benign cyst), and the day before my gynecological examination, I felt weak and dizzy. Several times I thought I was going to faint. My husband was out of town on a business trip. And that night, as I lay in bed alone and frightened, my fingers and toes began to feel ice cold and numb. The back of my head felt sore to the touch. I was shivering so much I had to put on an extra blanket. I became panic-stricken. I thought there was something terribly wrong with me. When I saw the doctor the next morning, he explained that I was hyperventilating, and that getting nervous about it only made me hyperventilate more. Whenever I felt that way, he said, I should breathe into

*a paper bag, or just cup my hands over my nose and mouth
and breathe into them."*

Stress can cause upset stomachs, headaches and sleep problems. If it is severe and prolonged enough it can eventually
affect a person's health. Stress has been linked to many physical illnesses, among them high blood pressure, stomach
ulcers, hormone imbalances and heart disease.[1]

How you cope with stress depends as much upon your personality as it does on external life events. Everyone has a different threshold level for stress. And the things that make one
person feel stressed may not affect another person at all.

If you are struggling with a problem, you may find it helpful
to keep the following general guidelines in mind:

• Focus only on the present, and only on aspects of the
problem that you have the power to change.

• Examine problems one at a time, and break them down
into manageable segments.

• Don't keep everything inside. Discuss your problems with
other people. Often family and friends can provide useful
suggestions.

• Don't sit and mull over it. Once you decide on a course
of action, take it.

Rating the Stresses in Your Life

To give you an idea of how stresses—both positive and negative—can combine to affect you, take a look at the *Social
Readjustment Rating Scale* that follows. It was devised by Drs.
Thomas H. Holmes and Richard H. Rahe in 1967, and shows
the relative impact of different events on our lives.[2] Holmes
and Rahe found that people who scored from 150 to 300 points
on this scale had a fifty-fifty chance of developing some type
of illness or health change within a year's time. Those who
scored over 300 had a 90 percent chance. As the score increases, the probability of a serious health change increases
as well.

The Social Readjustment Rating Scale*

Life Event	Mean Value
1. Death of spouse	100
2. Divorce	73
3. Marital separation from mate	65
4. Detention in jail or other institution	63
5. Death of a close family member	63
6. Major personal injury or illness	53
7. Marriage	50
8. Being fired at work	47
9. Marital reconciliation with mate	45
10. Retirement from work	45
11. Major change in health or behavior of a family member	44
12. Pregnancy	40
13. Sexual difficulties	39
14. Gaining a new family member (e.g., through birth, adoption, oldster moving in, etc.)	39
15. Major business readjustment (e.g., merger, reorganization, bankruptcy, etc.)	39
16. Major change in financial state (e.g., a lot worse off or a lot better off than usual)	38
17. Death of a close friend	37
18. Changing to a different line of work	36
19. Major change in the number of arguments with spouse (e.g., either a lot more or a lot less than usual regarding child-rearing, personal habits, etc.	35
20. Taking out a mortgage or loan for a major purchase (e.g., for a home, business, etc.)	31
21. Foreclosure on a mortgage or loan	30

The Social Readjustment Rating Scale (Continued)

Life Event	Mean Value
22. Major change in responsibilities at work (e.g., promotion, demotion, lateral transfer)	29
23. Son or daughter leaving home (e.g., marriage, attending college, etc.)	29
24. Trouble with in-laws	29
25. Outstanding personal achievement	28
26. Wife beginning or ceasing work outside the home	26
27. Beginning or ceasing formal schooling	26
28. Major change in living conditions (e.g., building a new home, remodeling, deterioration of home or neighborhood)	25
29. Revision of personal habits (dress, manners, associations, etc.)	24
30. Trouble with the boss	23
31. Major change in working hours or conditions	20
32. Change in residence	20
33. Changing to a new school	20
34. Major change in usual type and/or amount of recreation	19
35. Major change in church activities (e.g., a lot more or a lot less than usual)	19
36. Major change in social activities (e.g., clubs, dancing, movies, visiting, etc.)	18
37. Taking out a mortgage or loan for a lesser purchase (e.g., for a car, TV, freezer, etc.)	17
38. Major change in sleeping habits (a lot more or a lot less sleep, or change in part of day when asleep)	16

The Social Readjustment Rating Scale (Continued)

Life Event	Mean Value
39. Major change in number of family get-togethers (e.g., a lot more or a lot less than usual)	15
40. Major change in eating habits (a lot more or a lot less food intake, or very different meal hours or surroundings)	15
41. Vacation	13
42. Christmas	12
43. Minor violations of the law (e.g., traffic tickets, jaywalking, disturbing the peace, etc.)	11

Reprinted with permission from Journal of Psychosomatic Research, Vol. II, No. 2, Holmes, Thomas H. and Rahe, Richard H., "The Social Readjustment Rating Scale," copyright 1967, Pergamon Press, Ltd.

Stress Reduction Techniques That Help

You need not be at the total mercy of the stresses in your life. Stress reduction techniques can help you to get a handle on your emotions, and to "undo" the fight-or-flight response. They enable you to relax at will, and may be used any time and any place—whether it's in the gynecologist's examining room, before an important job interview or while you're having a hot flash. (In one recent study menopausal women were able to substantially reduce the number of their hot flashes after learning a variety of stress-reducing methods.[3])

If you have taken childbirth education classes in the past, you may already be familiar with some of the techniques that follow. Deep breathing and progressive relaxation have long been used to help relax women during labor.

The Jacobson Progressive Relaxation Technique

This technique teaches you how to systematically tense and then release individual muscles in your body. It was developed in the 1930s by Dr. Edmund Jacobson, and has been used in the treatment of insomnia, anxiety, obesity, heart disease, high blood pressure, indigestion, ulcers, colitis and phobias.

Explains one instructor: "When you are fully alert, it's as if your light switch is on. When you are relaxed, the switch is turned off. A tense person falls somewhere in between. His "switch" is stuck at the midway point. As he walks around with low-level tension it's as if his lights are flickering. The Jacobson Relaxation Technique exaggerates the relationship between tension and relaxation so that you can consciously turn the switch on and off whenever you want to."

Before practicing this, or any other relaxation techniques, find a quiet place where you won't be disturbed. Make sure that you are dressed comfortably, in loose-fitting clothes. Shoes should be loosened or kicked off, and eyeglasses removed. Do not practice too soon after a big meal, as the digestive processes can interfere with relaxation.

To begin, lie down on a soft quilt with your arms at your sides, or sit in a comfortable chair with your hands resting limply in your lap. Breathe in and out slowly, deeply and rhythmically. Notice how the inhaled breath causes tension and how the exhaled breath causes relaxation. When you feel relaxed, direct your attention to your feet. Tighten the muscles in one foot, hold for a few seconds, then relax. (Do not tighten your muscles to the point of discomfort or cramping.) Next, repeat with your other foot. Progress up your body, tightening and releasing muscles in each of your ankles, calves, knees and thighs. Tense and release muscles in your pelvic area, abdomen and buttocks. Then follow with each of your hands, forearms and upper arms. Don't rush hurriedly from muscle to muscle. Hold the tension for a few seconds and then slowly savor the relaxed feeling that comes from letting go. Relax your chest and lungs by taking a deep, slow, cleansing breath. Hunch your shoulders up to your ears, and then relax them. Bend your chin to your chest, and relax. Arch your back for a few moments, and then relax. Now focus on relaxing your jaw, eyelids, eyebrows, lips, forehead and scalp. Scrunch up your face, feeling all of the muscles in it, and then relax.

Your body by now should feel heavy, warm and limp from

head to toe. Take a mental inventory of your muscles, one by one. If any of them still feels tense, focus on sending a ripple of relaxation down toward it.

This exercise should be practiced for several minutes, twice a day.

The Relaxation Response

Herbert Benson, a cardiologist, popularized this technique in his book, *The Relaxation Response*. It is based upon methods used in transcendental meditation (TM). In TM, a person passively meditates on a secret "mantra" or syllable to help clear the mind of external thoughts. During meditation, practitioners are able to slow down their heart rates, respiration, blood pressure and overall metabolism.

Benson took the meditative aspects of TM, but stripped it of its spiritual meaning. He found that the repetition of any nonsense syllable could alter body states just as effectively as the repetition of a mantra. The syllable has to be a neutral one, without any disturbing associations. For many, the word "one" seems to work quite nicely.

To practice, deeply relax your muscles, progressing upward from your feet to your head. Keep them relaxed. Now focus on your breathing. Breathe slowly and naturally. Each time you exhale, you should feel more and more relaxed. With every breath out, silently say the word "one" or, if you prefer, just visually focus on the syllable. Your mind may tend to wander, but don't worry. Just say "oh, well" to yourself and return your attention to your breathing.

Benson recommends that you practice twice a day, for ten to twenty minutes at a time. (If you're a jogging enthusiast, you may want to incorporate this exercise into a portion of your run. Benson told one of his patients to do this by focusing on the "one-two" cadence of his footsteps.)

Creative Imagery

This technique is easy and fun. Simply close your eyes and picture, in minute detail, a scene that gives you a sense of peaceful repose. You can transport yourself to a cool, pine-scented forest, a hot sun-drenched beach, or even to a cabin in the woods, replete with crackling fireplace and a bearskin rug. During a hot flash you may want to conjure up an icy snow scene, or a cool forest glade. Use your senses of sight, taste, smell and sound to enter the scene in your mind's eye. It's your scene and you can embellish it to the hilt. You may develop three or four favorite fantasy spots that you'd like to return to in times of tension. Then, whenever you wish, simply close your eyes and take a mini-vacation from stress.

Mix and Match Techniques

At stress reduction workshops, instructors often combine some elements from each of the above techniques. So can you. Just pick and choose the aspects of each technique that relax you most effectively, and practice them daily.

The following is a summary of a blended method taught by instructors at an American Red Cross seminar.

Darken the room, close your eyes and breathe in and out, slowly and rhythmically. Repeat to yourself phrases like "I am," "Love," "Peace" or "One." After a few minutes, imagine that you are on an elevator that is decorated in any way that pleases you. (It may be lined with silk and have soft, fluffy cushions, or be of highly polished wood, or wrought iron.) The elevator begins to descend from the tenth floor. As it goes down and down, more deeply, you systematically relax each of your muscles beginning with your toes and working upward. (Think about each muscle becoming relaxed, heavy and limp, as if warm honey were oozing through your body.) By the time the elevator reaches the ground floor, you are in an entirely relaxed state.

The elevator door opens onto a beach. You step out and experience the scene. (Feel the warm sun on your skin and the grains of sand between your toes. See the billowy clouds ease across a perfectly blue sky. Listen to the crash of the waves. Smell the salt air and taste it on your lips.)

You come upon a beach blanket and lie down on it. Listen to the slow rhythm of your breath. Perhaps you drift off to sleep and dream that you are on a beach.

By the time you awaken, night has begun to fall. The sky is streaked with color. It is time to go. But first you take a barefoot run across the wet sand, or a swim in the salty ocean.

As you walk toward the elevator, you tell yourself that you feel strong, healthy and relaxed.

You begin the ascent, and as you rise you feel that each of your muscles (beginning at your head and working down to your toes) feels lighter. Your breathing, meanwhile, is rhythmic and relaxed. You arrive at the tenth floor and the elevator opens. Notice the sounds around you in the room. Gently stir your limbs. Open your eyes.

Some people feel warm or tingly after they perform their exercises. That's good. It means that you are deeply relaxing and that your blood is circulating freely. You are not, however, supposed to feel dizzy. That means that you are breathing too hard, and hyperventilating. You should stop practicing the exercise if you feel that way.

There are a number of other methods that effectively reduce tension levels, among them biofeedback, yoga and self-hypnosis. However, they require more formalized training and, in the case of biofeedback, expensive equipment.

Regular daily exercise is another excellent tension reliever. Ideas for setting up an exercise regimen that suits your needs will be discussed in Chapter 8.

Insomnia

Stress and insomnia often go hand in hand. Unresolved problems have a habit of popping up to the surface at night. Observes one insomniac: "As I toss and turn my worries march through my brain like an endless procession. There's my father who just had a heart attack, and my husband who is simply killing himself in the business he just started. I have my own job pressures. And my teenagers are a handful. Sometimes I feel as if my mind is on fire. But I can't stop the parade of worries no matter how I try." Night sweats may aggravate the problem, rousing a woman from a deep slumber only to leave her wide awake and unable to go back to sleep.

How do you know if you have insomnia? The following are some indications.

• If it takes you more than twenty or thirty minutes to fall asleep (it takes the average person fifteen minutes).

• If you find yourself using some sort of sleeping aid more than once or twice a week.

• If you awaken in the middle of the night and it takes you more than five or ten minutes to return to sleep again. (Most people awaken briefly several times each night, but the episodes are so brief that they are not usually recalled.)

Don't get riled just because you get less than eight hours of sleep a night. Eight hours is an ideal figure. Some people do very nicely on four hours a night while others feel groggy when they get fewer than nine. The key is not how many hours you sleep, but how you feel the next day.

Recognize, too, that the amount and quality of sleep changes as we age. A newborn baby may sleep as many as fourteen to eighteen hours a day, but adults usually need no more than seven or eight hours. As we continue to age our need for sleep decreases even further. And beginning at about age fifty the sleep we do get is lighter than it was before.[4] Many elderly people tend to sleep for a few hours in the evening and take an afternoon nap the following day.

Sleep needs also change according to our physical health and mental outlook. We need less sleep when we are feeling fit and happy, but more during times of illness, distress or depression.[5]

In experiments it has been observed that people often overestimate the time it actually takes them to get to sleep and underestimate the amount of sleep they actually get.[6] So although it sometimes feels as if you hardly slept a wink, you may, in actuality, have gotten more shut-eye than you suspect.

If you don't sleep well for a night or two, you'll be none the worse for wear in the long run. Observations of people who voluntarily stayed awake for several nights in a row show that one night of sound sleep can make up for the most severe sleep deprivation. A prolonged lack of sleep doesn't seem to interfere with tasks demanding highly developed skills; however, the performance of simple, boring routine tasks may be impaired.[7]

The stress reduction techniques previously described are excellent bedtime relaxants. They have been used successfully as sleep-inducing aids and are far safer than the repeated use of drugs or alcohol. Practice these methods first during the day, when you are not worrying about getting to sleep. Once you feel you have some mastery over them try them at night in bed, perhaps after a warm bath or shower.

"I used to be frantic about not getting enough sleep," says one woman. "Then I attended a stress reduction workshop, and learned a few techniques. Instead of lying awake with my mind drifting in and out of my daytime problems, I have a structure I can follow. I feel I have control over my mind rather than vice versa. By now I'm so good at relaxing that I start telling my toes to go to sleep, and by the time I reach the top of my head, I've already floated off. I never even make it to the visualization part."

The following tips should also prove helpful in coping with insomnia:

1. *Leave your worries outside of the bedroom door.* Worries make poor bed companions. If you have pressing problems set aside a special "worry time" earlier in the evening to think about them. The hour before bedtime should be reserved for unwinding. Soak in a hot bathtub, listen to soft music, read a pleasant book, or watch a relaxing TV program. Avoid any activity that is unpleasant or overly stimulating.

2. *Make sleep conditions comfortable.* If you've got a dripping faucet that's driving you crazy, or the street lamp outside glares in your eyes each time you roll over to your right side, do something about it. If you can't change the environment, then ear plugs or eye masks may prove helpful. Sleep on a firm, comfortable mattress. And keep the room at a comfortably cool temperature (between 62 and 66 degrees Fahrenheit).

Try to consciously perform a set series of bedtime rituals each night. This will condition your body to sleep. Most people perform such rituals automatically, when they brush their teeth, set the clock, shut the lights and pull down the covers.

3. *Get sufficient exercise.* Daily exercise makes for deeper sleep, and it's a good way of getting rid of excess tension. The best time to exercise is in the afternoon or early evening. Early morning exercise gives your body too much time to bounce back, and won't do anything to improve your sleep. Exercising

too close to bedtime can be overstimulating. The one exception to this rule is lovemaking, which seems to relieve tension and promote sleep. Masturbation, too, helps many people to drift off to sleep.

4. *Avoid evening stimulants.* Caffeine is a stimulant. It can speed up your pulse and respiration and give you the jitters. Some people develop an increased sensitivity to caffeine as they grow older. If you are having problems with insomnia it is best to avoid caffeine-containing substances, especially during late afternoon and early evening hours. This includes coffee, tea, cocoa, chocolate, and many soft drinks. Try substituting decaffeinated coffee; grain beverages, such as Postum or Cafix; herbal teas; carob candy or carob-powdered drinks (this is a vegetable-based product that looks and tastes remarkably like chocolate); juices and caffeine-free soft drinks. You may be surprised to know that caffeine is present in many over-the-counter cold pills, pain relievers and diet pills. (See accompanying chart.) As a general rule, more than 250 mg. of caffeine consumed within six hours of bedtime can disturb sleep.[8]

Cigarette smoke is another stimulant that can interfere with sleep, and heavy smokers may find that they are roused easily in the middle of the night.[9] Add this to your arsenal of reasons to quit the habit.

5. *Try some sensible sleep remedies.* An occasional glass of wine may help put you to sleep. In the long run, however, alcohol is a poor nightcap. It suppresses REM and delta sleep—the deeper, more rejuvenating sleep stages—so that alcohol-induced slumber tends to be lighter and less refreshing. You eventually need larger and larger amounts of alcohol for it to have the same effects.

Be wary, too, of sleeping pills. They may be helpful in times of extreme stress. But don't get into the habit of using them nightly. They are only effective for a short while (usually about two weeks) and then the dosage has to be upped in order to get the same effect. As with alcohol, the kind of sleep resulting from pills is lighter and more fragmented than normal. And they may leave you feeling groggy in the morning. With regular use, the body becomes dependent upon sleeping pills. When they are stopped there may be a withdrawal effect, in-

Caffeine Content of Beverages, Foods and Drugs

Item	Milligrams Caffeine
Coffee (5-oz. cup)	
Brewed, drip method	60–180
Brewed, percolator	40–170
Instant	30–120
Decaffeinated, brewed	2–5
Decaffeinated, instant	1–5
Tea (5-oz. cup)	
Brewed, major U.S. brands	20–90
Brewed, imported brands	25–110
Instant	25–50
Iced (12-oz. glass)	67–76
Cocoa beverage (5-oz. cup)	2–20
Chocolate milk beverage (8 oz.)	2–7
Milk chocolate (1 oz.)	1–15
Dark chocolate, semi-sweet (1 oz.)	5–35
Baker's chocolate (1 oz.)	26
Chocolate-flavored syrup (1 oz.)	4
Cola Drinks (12 oz.)	30–59

Source: FDA, Food Additive Chemistry Evaluation Branch, based on evaluations of existing literature on caffeine levels.

Prescription Drugs

Cafergot (for migraine headache)	100
Fiorinal (for tension headache)	40
Soma Compound (pain relief, muscle relaxant)	32
Darvon Compound (pain relief)	32.4

Caffeine Content of Beverages, Foods and Drugs

Item	Milligrams Caffeine
Nonprescription Drugs	
Weight-Control Aids	
Dex-A-Diet II	200
Dexatrim, Dexatrim Extra Strength	200
Dietac capsules	200
Maximum Strength Appedrine	100
Prolamine	140
Alertness Tablets	
Nodoz	100
Vivarin	200
Analgesic/Pain Relief	
Anacin, Maximum Strength Anacin	32
Excedrin	65
Midol	32.4
Vanquish	33
Diuretics	
Aqua-Ban	100
Maximum Strength Aqua-Ban Plus	200
Permathene H2 Off	200
Cold/Allergy Remedies	
Coryban-D capsules	30
Triaminicin tablets	30
Dristan Decongestant tablets and Dristan A-F Decongestant tablets	16.2
Duradyne-Forte	30

Source: FDA's National Center for Drugs and Biologics.
Reprinted from FDA Consumer, 1984

cluding sleeplessness, irritability, anxiety and vivid nightmares.

Dalmane is currently the most widely used of the prescription sleeping pills. It is longer-lasting than the other barbiturates (effective for up to one month) and it is less addictive. However, it does reduce the deeper stages of sleep so that a person using Dalmane may feel fatigued and out of sorts the following day—the very problem which insomniacs are trying to avoid.[10]

Try topping the evening off with a glass of warm milk or Ovaltine. These substances contain tryptophan—a naturally occurring amino acid that induces sleep. Tryptophan is also found in meat, poultry, soybeans and dairy products, which explains why people so often feel sleepy after a large meal. Tryptophan is available in tablet form from health food stores and pharmacies.

A hot cup of herbal tea can be soothing before bedtime. Herbs such as chamomile, scullcap, valerian root, hops, passion flower and rosehips are especially good for calming the nerves, according to one health food store manager. Some women also find mint tea to be relaxing. (In her book *Hygiea: A Woman's Herbal*, Jeannine Parvati reports that the smell of the herb hops, used in the production of beer, can be sleep-inducing, and that some can be tucked inside your pillow for a calmative effect.) If you wish, you may visit a health food store and have a blend of herbs specially prepared for your needs. One commercially available tea called Sleepytime already includes several of the above-mentioned herbs.

Have a cracker or slice of cheese with your milk or herbal tea. A *light* snack at bedtime seems to encourage sound sleep.

6. *Use your bed for sleeping only.* When you think bedroom, think sleep. The only two activities that should be reserved for the bedroom are sleep and sex. If you want to watch TV, read a book, balance your checkbook, or squabble with your spouse—do it elsewhere. Your bedroom should never be associated with these stimulating activities.

7. *Keep sleep habits regular.* The longer the time interval before you go to bed, the easier it is to fall asleep. So, if you have a problem with insomnia, it is best to avoid daytime naps. Set your alarm clock for the same time each day, seven days

a week. That way you'll help your body learn to feel tired at about the same time each night. And don't go to bed until you're really sleepy—no matter what the clock dial reads. Trying to sleep when your body is still in full gear will only heighten your anxiety at bedtime.

8. *If you are having trouble sleeping . . .* Give yourself a good fifteen to twenty minutes to fall asleep and then—if all seems futile—get up and out of the bedroom. It serves no purpose to thrash around between the sheets. Instead, perform some low-keyed activity, like folding laundry, sewing, writing the week's menus out or reading through an encyclopedia. Return to bed only when you feel sleepy, and repeat the procedure as many times as necessary.

If you awaken in the middle of the night, try not to rouse yourself too much. In the case of night sweats, keep a fresh nighty at hand's reach so that you may change in the dark, without having to get up out of bed. Take a mental inventory of your muscles from toe to head telling yourself that they are warm, heavy and so deeply relaxed that you cannot even move them. "I keep my clock facing to the wall," says one woman who has had a bout with night wakings. "That way I'm not tempted to glance at the clock and upset myself by seeing what time it is and how many hours I have left until I have to get up for work." If you do awaken fully and stay awake longer than fifteen or twenty minutes, go into another room and do some nonstimulating activity until you feel sleepy.

Early risers sometimes confuse a decreased need for sleep with insomnia. If after five or six hours of sleep you awaken, raring to go, then that's probably all of the sleep your body needs. There's no reason to continue lying there, forcing yourself to get extra hours of sleep. Instead, get up and start the day.

9. *Seek help when it's needed.* Try not to worry yourself sick over lack of sleep. Your body knows when it's tired and will naturally give itself up to rest when you need it. No permanent harm will come to you from several nights of disturbed slumber.

If, however, you feel that sleep disturbances are becoming an overwhelming problem in your life, you may want to seek professional help, beginning with a physical examination to rule out other possible health problems. In the case of severe, persistent night sweats, your physician may want to prescribe estrogen. This often provides prompt relief and allows a woman to get a good night's rest.

Sleep clinics, which specialize in the study of sleep disturbances, may be of help in other instances of severe insomnia. To contact the sleep center nearest you call the psychiatric department at your local medical school or hospital, or write to the address at the end of this book.

Menopause Support Groups

It is far healthier to talk to other people about your problems than it is to keep them bottled up inside: "I belong to a bridge club," says one fifty-eight-year-old, "but over the many years we've been meeting it's really become a therapy group as well. We talk about problems we've had with our husbands and children. Several of us have gone through menopause at about the same time. It is interesting to see how differently each of us has experienced it." A supportive husband and sympathetic family and friends can do wonders for putting problems into their proper perspective.

One positive outgrowth of the women's movement has been the popularization of support groups—women who get together to share common joys, frustrations and concerns. Since the 1960s, when consciousness raising groups were in vogue, the support group concept has mushroomed. Today women meet in groups to discuss all kinds of special issues from parenting, to self-help health care, to menopause.

"The women who attend my menopause support groups inevitably say that the experience is terrific and that they are so glad to be sharing their feelings," reports one nurse and menopause group facilitator. Says a group participant: "I couldn't believe that other women were feeling the exact same way I was. It was great!"

You may feel funny about joining a support group if you've never been in one before. How will you have the nerve to talk about personal things in front of so many strangers? Most everyone feels a bit apprehensive at first. But the dynamics of support groups are such that strangers quickly grow to be friends.

To find a menopause support group in your area, inquire at your local YMCA, YWCA, women's groups, department of health, Planned Parenthood, family or community health agencies, the American Red Cross, colleges, hospitals, temples or churches. If these organizations do not already have an ongoing group, they may be able to direct you to one. Some agencies are willing to set up a group for you so long as you can demonstrate that there is a community need for it. At the very least, ask if they are willing to provide you with a meeting place and if they will allow you to use their bulletin board or agency newsletter to recruit potential group members.

You do not necessarily need the help of an agency to form a support group. Many women meet informally in each other's homes on a rotating basis. Such informal support groups can be formed by anyone, any time. If you'd like to form one yourself, here are a few guidelines.

• Keep the group small—anywhere from eight to twelve women. That way you'll be able to maintain a feeling of intimacy and give all a chance to participate. The group may be open to anyone who shares concerns about menopause, from the thirty-eight-year-old whose periods are becoming irregular to the sixty-year-old who wonders whether she should continue to stay on estrogen therapy.

• Choose a group facilitator. This should preferably be someone who has had some experience in leading groups. The facilitator's role is to gently guide discussions so that they don't get bogged down, and so that everyone has an equal chance to speak.

• Make a time commitment. Plan to meet weekly for three to five sessions. A short-term commitment is easier for women to agree to. After the predetermined time has elapsed, you can vote on whether or not there is a need to extend the group.

• Strict confidentiality should be the rule. Women should agree ahead of time that all conversations are private, and not to be repeated outside of the group.

What will you discuss at each meeting? Every support group will find that it has its own unique concerns and needs. The following is a list of suggested topics. It was adapted, in part, from guidelines set forth by The Menopause Collective in Cambridge, Massachusetts.[11] You may use them as a springboard in creating your own agenda.

Meeting 1: Introductions
Begin by going around in a circle as each participant introduces herself and tells why she came to the group. Feelings about menstruation and menopause may be explored by asking the following questions: How did you feel when you first got your period? Did your mother prepare you for it? What was her attitude toward menstruation? What was your mother's menopause like? Did she discuss it with you? How do you feel about going through menopause? Leave time for women to discuss the topics they would like to see covered in subsequent meetings. Each person can take one of the topics to read up on and present at a later date. Chapters plus suggested readings from this book might form the basis for discussions. (Make sure your research materials are up-to-date. Knowledge about menopause has changed dramatically in the past decade or two!)

Meeting 2: The Symptoms of Menopause
What are the symptoms of menopause? (Changes in menstrual cycles, hot flashes, night sweats, vaginal dryness.) What causes these symptoms? Have you experienced any of them? How do they feel? Has anything you've done helped to alleviate them? Are you: taking estrogen, vitamins, herbs, exercising? Have you changed your eating habits? Do you experience more exaggerated mood swings, nervousness, irritability, dizziness, palpitations, tingling or numbness of the extremities? When? What do you do to cope? What is the difference between natural and surgical menopause?

Meeting 3: Menopause vs. Aging
How is menopause different from aging? Have you experienced any noticeable physical or health changes as you've aged? (Weight gain, changes in skin and hair texture, wrinkles,

graying, arthritis, etc.) How do you think society views the aging female (talk about roles of middle-aged women in movies, books, television)? How do you feel about the lack of periods and the end of the childbearing role? Has menopause affected you as a sexual person? Do men also change emotionally, physically and sexually as they age?

Meeting No. 4: Positive Aspects of the Middle Years
What are some of the positive aspects about menopause and growing older? (E.g., growth in self-confidence, more free time, no more worries about pregnancy.) What are some of the losses that you may face? (E.g., death of parents, grown children leaving home, divorce, widowhood.) Who were the most important middle-aged women in your life? What special qualities did they have? Name some positive female role models in politics, movies, TV, literature. What are your long-range plans for the next thirty years? (E.g., back to work, back to school, retirement, etc.)

You may or may not want to extend the group meetings at this point. If you do, discuss a possible future agenda based on issues not yet covered.

Some support groups arrange to have professional speakers to kick off their meetings. Often physicians, nurses, nutritionists, psychologists, career counselors and other experts will give lectures to interested community groups. Some provide the service for free, while others charge a fee. If you do have a guest speaker be sure to schedule ample time for group discussion and questions—women should have an opportunity to talk at each session.

Professional Counseling

Friendly advice, relaxation techniques and support groups can be a great help in coping with mid-life ups and downs. "However," cautions one professional counselor, "they may only be like Band-aids when a woman's emotional problems are severe." If she is feeling so overwhelmed by depression, guilt and low self-esteem that she cannot function on a day-to-day basis, then professional counseling may be in order.

How do you go about finding a professional therapist? If you have friends or relatives who have had a good experience with therapy you might ask them for a reference. Your family doctor, clergy and local mental health association are other good sources for referrals. You might call the head of the psychiatry department at the medical school or hospital nearest you and ask him or her for a recommendation.

Therapists come from different schools of thought and take different approaches to treatment. It's important that you have good rapport with the one you select. You may have to do a bit of footwork—including one or two initial therapy sessions—before you settle on the therapy situation that's right for you.

Reentering the Job Market

Working is good for your health. At least that's the consensus reached in several studies done on the subject. Middle-aged women with outside jobs appear to be in better physical health and to have more self-esteem than their stay-at-home counterparts. They also appear to pass through menopause with the least number of complaints. The women who have the most difficulties at menopause are typically housewives with little interest outside of their homes and families. [12,13,14]

While going back to work may be good for you, it is not always an easy step to take. How do you account for a ten- or twenty-year gap in your resume? What if you've never had any work experience at all? Self-confidence often dwindles in the face of rusty work skills. Reflects one homemaker: "What do I want? It's a hard question for a middle-aged woman. Can I give mothering up? Will I be good at other things?"

Luckily, there's a trend afoot to assist displaced homemakers. More career and educational opportunities are available to women in their middle years than ever before. Career counseling services and job-reentry programs are springing up throughout the country.

If you think you need the services of a career counselor, you might start by writing to Catalyst, a national, nonprofit organization based in New York City. Catalyst exists solely to promote women in the work force. They have a national referral service, and can direct you to career counseling and continuing education programs in localities across the country. (For information, write to them at the address at the back of this book.)

Most career counseling centers offer a three-part program: 1) Self-evaluation exercises, to help you figure out what your skills and interests are. 2) Research into possible careers. 3) Job-hunting techniques, including how to write a resume and conduct yourself at a job interview. Some programs have internships, where you can gain work experience as an unsalaried apprentice in your chosen field.

Back-to-Work Hurdles

The amount of difficulty a woman may have in reentering the job market will depend upon her educational level, her job history, and the type of employment she had before she dropped out of the work force. Says one women's career counselor: "Some women chose to stay home because it was important to them to be there for their kids. But at the same time they were the movers and the shakers of their community. They identified needs in their neighborhoods and took action to initiate changes. They've had an ongoing engagement in the world. And they can take these skills and utilize them on a resume and in job interviews. The woman who was mainly a homemaker may have more of a struggle. Society doesn't value the role of homemakers. So we have to work on building her self-esteem and on making her aware that she does have marketable skills."

A middle-aged woman may see her age and lack of paid work experience as major hurdles. But they needn't be. The expertise needed to run a home, balance the family budget, and serve on school, religious and civic committees may translate into valuable work skills. Sometimes it's simply a matter of knowing how to highlight your skills in a resume. If you have large gaps in your salaried job history, for example, you may want to use a functional resume instead of a standard chronological one. In the functional resume, your experience is listed under subject headings such as "Management Experience," or "Public Relations Skills," rather than by date or company. "The idea is to pique your potential employer's interest before he or she gets to the references," says this same counselor.

"Always know ahead of time how you are going to handle the most problematic questions that might arise at a job interview and turn them into positives," she adds. If you think your age will be viewed as a possible liability, be prepared to convince your potential employer that it is, in fact, a valuable asset: You are mature and stable. You are an eager learner and are enthusiastic about taking on this new job. You won't be taking maternity leave, or having to juggle your work time with the needs of young children. And you intend to devote many productive years to your job. Younger women just out of school or raising young families cannot offer the same attributes.

One forty-three-year-old biology teacher tells how she was able to reenter the job market after first being rebuffed on many interviews: "I was good at teaching, but I didn't like the role. When I was ready to go back to work I knew I wanted to do something else. So I went back to school and studied for my master's in counseling. After I got my degree, I went on a job search, and did I ever feel old. I was interviewed by men who were unsympathetic toward me. In each case a kid in his twenties was hired and not me. I was seen as too old for an entry-level position. My skills and education were not valued at all. So I went to a career placement center for advice. The counselor said that I should stress to my employer what a bargain he was getting. That I have all of the skills for the entry-level position, and that I was more than willing and able to do the work. In addition, they'd be gaining because I can make extra contributions based upon my previous skills, experience and training. I never thought to approach it that way. I eventually landed a job as a guidance counselor."

There are many helpful books available on job searching, and several are listed in the back of this book.

Volunteer Work

If you don't have to work out of financial necessity and are apprehensive about competing in the job market, you might want to consider a volunteer job. Volunteer work can be a stepping stone to paid employment, or it can be a satisfying way to spend extra hours in your day. For many it is a confidence-builder, as well as a way of acquiring new skills.

One woman who had a flair for writing volunteered to do public relations work for a short-staffed community center: "At first I helped to write and proofread the agency's newsletter. After a while they asked me to write an occasional brochure and press release. When a salaried position became available, I was offered the job." Another, who was interested in women's health issues, volunteered to work for Planned Parenthood: "They put me in an intensive volunteer training program, and soon I was off giving talks and slide presentations on rape prevention to groups throughout the community. I developed a poise and confidence I never knew I had. It has been a tremendous learning experience."

Volunteer work can be a great outlet for the woman who misses nurturing young children at home: "I always loved little children. So when my kids were out of the house, I volunteered to work at the children's hospital. I read to the kids, and play with them, and make them feel a little less sad that they're away from their mommies. It makes me feel like I'm really doing something worthwhile with my life." The woman who enjoys being around youngsters might also want to consider foster child programs, or helping out in day-care centers, schools or mental health centers.

To get an idea of what agencies might need your skills, visit your local library. Most of them keep a directory of local associations in their reference department. You might also get ideas by thumbing through different subject headings, such as "Associations" or "Social Service Organizations" in the Yellow Pages of your phone book.

Choosing to Stay at Home

Some women feel socially pressured to reenter the job market even though it's something they do not really need or want to do. One job counselor offers this anecdote:

"About a year ago Beth came to the career center. She needed help in changing her career. She was a former home economics teacher. But she decided to work only part-time, as a substitute teacher, while her children were growing up. Now one of her children was a college senior and the other was in high school. Beth spent eight months doing intensive research on job searching but nothing 'clicked.' When asked what was important to her, she mentioned her home, her relationship with her husband and her time (much of which she spent designing and sewing clothes). Where did she want to go in her life? TV and the experts told her that to stay at home wasn't trendy. But when we probed a bit further we discovered that what Beth really wanted was to stay home. Now that she has explored her own desires she's content about her decision, as opposed to the woman biting her nails because she had no job. She had assumed that the media's needs were her own."

It is unfair to label homemakers as bored or unfulfilled. Civic involvement, hobbies, sports and personal interests can keep a woman's life full and interesting. A paycheck is not the only measure of self-worth.

A Matter of Choice

There are so many choices facing a woman in her middle years today: Should she return to work? Change careers? Go back to school? Work full-time or part-time? Remain a homemaker? The decision-making process can sometimes be a bewildering one:

"I gave up my job as a nursery-school teacher. I had begun writing a book and wanted to turn to it full-time. But working at home made me feel isolated and depressed. I thought maybe of becoming an occupational therapist. That's an area that always interested me. But it requires a lot of retraining and long hours. I don't want to sacrifice my family life for my job goals. I heard about a job opening in the public relations department of a museum. I've published a few articles in the local paper and am good at writing. I almost applied for it, but my stomach tied up in knots at the thought. At this point I'm not sure exactly what I want to do with the rest of my life."

Perhaps life was simpler in generations past, when women's

roles were more well-defined. But it couldn't have been more exciting. For the first time in history, it can truly be said that life begins at forty. Women are having fewer children and living longer. That means that they have many productive years left after their last child leaves home. What you choose to do with these years is up to you. There are many possibilities. And if the decision-making process is stressful, it may also be invigorating.

"I was a homemaker all of my married life. Then, when the kids were teenagers, my husband started his own business. He asked me to help him run it. I was a little uptight about it at first. I had little business experience, and I didn't know how it would be to work so closely with my husband all day long. It turned out to be the best thing that ever happened to me. I'm the one that deals with the clients best. And it's me who goes flying all around the country to give product presentations. I'm glad the days of cub scouts and PTA are past me. I just love getting out there meeting people. I'm thriving on it. This is the best time of my life."

A person may describe a glass of water as half empty or half full depending on his outlook. The same can be said of the woman who stands at the midpoint of her life. She may see her middle years as a life half over. Or she may see it as a unique time in which to explore new possibilities and set new goals.

Chapter 6
Estrogen
Therapy:
Yes or No?

"**I** don't like taking pills of any kind. In fact, I won't even take aspirin unless the need is extreme. I decided I'd rather suffer through the flashes than subject myself to hormones, and maybe to cancer."—Age fifty-three.

"I'll take estrogen until I die—or if I develop breast cancer. I plan to keep skiing well into my old age and don't want my bones to get brittle, or my hips to break."—Age fifty-eight.

"As an administrator, I had to lecture in front of large groups of people. It was mortifying to flush and perspire so much in the midst of a talk. Finally, I went to the doctor and he put me on estrogen. The relief was immediate. It was just wonderful. I stayed on estrogen for a few years and then went off it. I still get hot flashes once in a while, but not the way I used to."—Age sixty.

"*I went on estrogen for flashes and night sweats. It didn't help at all, and it made me very tired and lifeless. I have decided to suffer without it.*"—Age fifty-two.

"*I started estrogen therapy twenty-five years ago, after a hysterectomy for a fibroid tumor. My doctor retired and the new doctor said he thought I could do without the estrogen at my age. I stopped taking it for six weeks, but I went into a deep depression, like I never had before. So I started on the estrogen again and immediately felt better. When I told the doctor, his attitude was: 'Oh, well, if you think it's helping you there's probably no harm in your continuing to take it.'*"—Age seventy-six.

"*Estrogen gave me such terrible pains in the back of my head that I couldn't even lay my head down on a pillow. I decided to bear with the flashes instead. At this stage, they hardly ever bother me anymore.*"—Age sixty-three.

"*I had a total hysterectomy when I was in my late twenties. The doctor said that I might feel uncomfortable, and if I did, he would prescribe something for me. What an understatement! My emotional self went way out of sorts. Like having premenstrual blahs and bloats, but five times as bad. I couldn't get a grip on myself. Then I began to get the flashes—though at the time I didn't know that was what they were. It was like someone was filling me with hot liquid, starting at my feet and reaching up to my hairline. Then I'd get the chills and shakes. My husband thought it was a psychological change, that I was going nutty because I lost my uterus. Finally, I called the doctor and got a prescription for estrogen. Now I swear by it. It gives me some side effects—like nausea and headaches—but it takes away the flashes and keeps me even-keeled.*"—Age thirty-three.

"*The people who tell you not to take estrogen really anger me. They're not the ones flapping around all night with the sweats. They don't know what it feels like to have a dry vagina. My vagina was so painful that I could hardly move. It was killing my sex life and my marriage. I took estrogen pills for two years. And now I still use vaginal cream occasionally. It has restored my life to normal."—Age sixty.*

The great majority of women pass through menopause without seeking medical care. But an estimated fifteen to twenty-five percent ask their doctors for medical advice on coping with symptoms.[1] The only drug known to reliably relieve menopausal discomforts is estrogen. And a woman may have to decide whether or not to begin a hormone regimen which may last months, years or even a lifetime.

As a good medical consumer you should learn all that you can about the pros and cons of estrogen therapy before taking it. But there is so much conflicting information published about hormone treatment for menopause. Physicians themselves disagree as to who should and should not take hormones, and for how long. In the view of one gynecologist in private practice: "Women living past their reproductive function are a modern phenomenon, and the ovary is the only endocrinologic organ that poops out in total. I believe that the estrogen has to be replaced, and that women need to be on hormone therapy for life. Wouldn't we give therapy if the thyroid suddenly stopped functioning?" Another gynecologist disputes this view: "Not all women need replacement therapy. Only those with severe problems or at high risk for osteoporosis. What we do need is an improved way of identifying those women at risk."

The "Birth" of Estrogen Therapy

The reason that there is so much disagreement about estrogen therapy is that the study of menopause is still relatively young. Before the twentieth century, physicians thought that hot flashes and other menopausal symptoms had something to do with the retention of menstrual blood. Women were bled, leeched and given laxatives in an effort to purge their bodies of menstrual impurities. Their ovaries were surgically removed, and rest cures were prescribed in the hope of curing an assortment of sexual and nervous disorders, all attributed to menopause.

The twentieth century brought a new understanding of the

relationship between ovaries and sex hormones. Estrogen therapy was officially born in 1929 when Adolf Butenandt, a Nobel prize–winning chemist, isolated the hormone in the urine of pregnant women. But the use of estrogens for treating menopausal symptoms did not become widespread until 1966, when Brooklyn gynecologist Robert Wilson published his blockbuster book, *Feminine Forever.*

Wilson painted an incredibly grim portrait of menopause, calling it a "horror of . . . living decay."[2] He then went on to make many extravagant claims for hormone treatment. It would cure menopause, he said, much as insulin cures diabetes. With hormones a woman could retain her supple figure and smooth skin and remain forever feminine. He advised women to start on estrogen treatment *before* the ravages of menopause began, and to continue taking it until the grave.

The news of a fountain of youth sent women stampeding to the bookstores and to their physicians. Articles in *Look* and *Vogue* added fuel to the fire, as did aggressive advertising campaigns in medical journals (much of Wilson's research was funded by the pharmaceutical industry). One hundred thousand copies of *Feminine Forever* were sold within seven months of publication. And the sale of estrogen quadrupled by 1975. Estrogen became the fourth or fifth most commonly prescribed drug in the United States.[3]

Then something happened to put a damper on this estrogen euphoria. In 1975 several independent research teams showed that women who were treated with estrogens for over a year had an increased risk of developing endometrial cancer (cancer of the lining of the uterus). The longer a woman stayed on estrogen therapy the greater her chances for developing this cancer.

Soon after, the Federal Drug Administration sent a bulletin to physicians which warned them of the link between endometrial cancer and estrogen use. The FDA recommended that estrogens be used in the lowest possible dose for the shortest possible time. By 1978 a law was passed requiring that estrogen-containing drugs include a patient insert clearly explaining the risks of therapy. In light of the new FDA warnings, estrogen usage declined by 40 percent.[4]

Today, most physicians take a conservative approach to estrogen therapy, recommending it only for severe and life-disrupting symptoms. When administered properly, with appropriate follow-up care, estrogen is still felt to be a valuable tool. "Unfortunately," says one gynecologist, "the fantasy of consumer protection has been replaced by consumer fear. I think that women now are unduly frightened of estrogen therapy."

Approximately 10 to 14 percent of all American women over forty-five are currently taking estrogen.[5,6]

What Estrogen Can and Cannot Do

Wilson claimed that estrogen was an age-defying drug capable of curing dozens of menopausal symptoms. Present claims for estrogen are less grandiose. The general medical consensus is that estrogen therapy is effective in the relief of *only two major menopausal symptoms*: hot flashes and vaginal atrophy (a thinning of the vaginal lining which can lead to irritation, painful intercourse and sometimes urinary tract problems). Estrogen has also been found to help prevent osteoporosis, the bone-thinning disease that can result in fractures in later life.

The use of estrogens for "nervous" symptoms is still controversial. As we've mentioned earlier, hot flashes and night sweats can play havoc with a woman's psyche. So can a dry, painful vagina that makes sexual intercourse uncomfortable or impossible. By clearing up these symptoms estrogen may indirectly improve a woman's mental outlook.

Physicians are less certain about whether depression alone—in the absence of flashes or vaginal atrophy—is reason enough to give a woman estrogen therapy. It is generally thought that relaxation techniques, counseling and perhaps antidepressant drugs are a better approach (see Chapter 5 for a more complete discussion).

Some researchers believe that estrogen may help to clear up insomnia, if this problem begins suddenly at menopause. In studies, the hormone has increased the REM (dream) stage of sleep in menopausal women. Again, it's not clear whether the sleep improvement was due to the hormone itself, or to the overall tonic effect that comes when estrogen clears up night sweats.[7,8,9]

One thing is certain: estrogen is not a magical cure for advancing age. Wrinkles, sagging skin and a redistribution of weight around the middle will come, with estrogen or without it. There is some slight evidence that estrogen may give breasts and skin a fuller look. But this needs further documentation.[10,11] Most experts agree that the cosmetic improvement (if, indeed, there is any) is not a sufficient reason to go on a hormone regimen. Exercise, a nutritional diet and an active mind are the real keys to growing older with health and grace.

In a 1981 meeting, experts at the World Health Organization surveyed 383 scientific references on menopause and came to this conclusion: Menopause is a natural part of aging and no treatment is necessary unless a specific disease or symptoms need to be treated or prevented.[12]

Endometrial Cancer

Though endometrial cancer is a relatively uncommon disease (it normally occurs in one woman in a thousand per year), its incidence soared in eight different regions in the country between the mid-sixties and seventies. This rise coincided with the publication of *Feminine Forever*.[13]

The link between uterine cancer and estrogen use is now undisputed. Women who take estrogen for two to four years are found to be at least four to eight times more likely to develop this disease. The risks increase the longer a woman is on estrogen therapy and when higher doses are taken.[14] It is widely believed that when a woman goes off estrogen therapy, her chances for developing endometrial cancer drop down to where they were before.[15] However, one new study found the risks of endometrial cancer to be significantly higher than usual, even ten years after women had stopped using estrogen.[16]

The reason that estrogen increases the risk of endometrial cancer is that it stimulates the uterus to build up a lining. During the reproductive years, such a lining would normally be sloughed off at menstruation. But the menopausal woman doesn't have monthly periods. The effects of estrogen on her uterus are unopposed. That is, they are not being counteracted by the second hormone in the menstrual cycle—progesterone. In some cases, the buildup of cells on the uterine lining becomes excessive, and develops into a condition known as hyperplasia. Hyperplasia can lead to cancer and is considered a strong reason for hysterectomy.

Doctors are reluctant to give estrogen therapy to obese women because they are already at high risk for developing cancer of the uterus. The body's main source of estrogen after menopause is from conversion of a male hormone in the fat cells of a woman's body (see Chapter 2, The Female Hormones). Obese women have more fat cells, and therefore higher levels of estrogen circulating in their bodies after menopause. They are less likely to have hot flashes or osteoporosis than their thinner sisters. At the same time, the estrogen they produce is unopposed by progesterone and makes them more likely targets for endometrial cancer. Women twenty-five to fifty pounds overweight have three times the normal rate of uterine cancer and women over fifty pounds overweight have a ninefold increase.[17]

Fortunately, the type of cancer produced by estrogen therapy is a less severe form than that which occurs naturally. It has a very high cure rate (90 to 95 percent). Although the number of cases of endometrial cancer rose in this country, the number of deaths from it did not.[18]

Many more precautions are taken today to prevent women on estrogen therapy from developing endometrial cancer. Estrogen is given in lower doses now, and for shorter periods of time. It is also given cyclically, rather than continuously, so that a woman's body has a drug-free week each month in which to rest. Doctors are also trying to mimic the natural menstrual cycle by adding a synthetic form of progesterone to the estrogen therapy. One widely publicized study at the Wilford Hall USAF Medical Center showed that women on low-dose estrogen-progesterone therapy for seven years had an even lower incidence of endometrial cancer than non-estrogen users.[19] It seems possible that the added progesterone has a protective effect against endometrial cancer for some women.

Breast Cancer

The tissue in a woman's breasts is similar to the tissue that lines her uterus. Both are sensitive to changes in female sex hormones. Though breast cells don't build up and shed monthly as do the cells of the uterine lining, cystic and abnormal cell growth changes in breast tissue have been shown by breast mammography to occur after estrogen therapy is started. These changes reverse themselves when a woman stops taking estrogen.[20]

Since high-dose, long-term use of estrogen can cause cancer of the uterus, there is some concern that it might cause breast cancer too. A link between estrogen and breast cancer has been found in experiments with animals. But studies on women do not yield any consistent conclusions. Some researchers have found an increase in breast cancer among estrogen users (usually those having it continuously at high doses on a long-term basis). Others have found no link at all. Women who have been on long-term oral contraceptives containing estrogen and progesterone do not have higher breast cancer rates.

Physicians simply do not know as much about breast cancer as they do about endometrial cancer. The disease appears to have many causes, including heredity, viruses, environment and hormones. In addition, it takes a very long time for breast cancers to develop—anywhere from ten to twenty years, and sometimes more. So far the rate of breast cancer cases among the general population has remained pretty stable over the last several decades, despite an increase in the use of estrogens.[21] But at this point we still may not be seeing the full story.

It is thought that estrogen may accelerate the growth of existing breast tumors. But whether or not it can cause a cancer to start is unknown.[22] To play it safe, physicians do not recommend estrogen therapy for women with a history of breast cancer or benign breast disease.

In the seven-year study at Wilford Hall USAF Medical Center, the women on a combination estrogen-progesterone therapy had lower breast cancer rates than either women who were using estrogen alone, or those who did not take any hormones at all.[23] So the added progesterone may protect the breasts as well as the uterus from cancer. (The long-term risks of progesterone are still being studied, and it does have some risks of its own, as we shall see later.)

Heart Disease

Women in this country have a lower incidence of heart disease than men. Then, sometime around menopause, this female advantage is lost. Scientists aren't sure exactly why this happens. They suspect that declining estrogen levels may play a role.

At menopause there is a dramatic change in the types of lipoproteins in a woman's blood (the proteins that carry fat through the blood). There is a drop in the number of high density lipoproteins, or HDLs, the "good guys" who sweep away fatty substances so that they do not accumulate on the walls of the arteries. And there is a rise in low density lipoproteins, or LDLs, the "bad guys" who encourage fatty deposits to occur. The new HDL/LDL balance favors the development of hardening of the arteries (atherosclerosis) and heart attacks. Estrogen therapy seems to partially reverse this profile, moving it back in a healthier direction.[24]

Autopsies done on women who have had a surgical menopause at an early age (both ovaries removed) show that the earlier the hysterectomy was done, the more fatty deposits there were on the artery walls. Advanced atherosclerosis was seen more often in women who were not treated with estrogen than in those who were.[25,26,27] These findings bolster the theory that falling estrogen levels may contribute to heart disease.

Heart disease, like breast cancer, may have many contributing causes, including diet, heredity, smoking, alcohol and stress. So it would be foolish to point an accusing finger at falling estrogen levels alone. And consider this curious riddle: while the ratio of male/female death rates from heart disease is high in the U.S., the disparity is not so great in other countries. In the 1950s, for example, when male/female death rates from heart disease in the U.S. were 5:1 among individuals aged forty-five to fifty-four, it was 2:1 in Italy and only 1:1 in Japan. Maybe the whole premise that heart disease accelerates in women after menopause is a false one. According to some researchers, it may just be that a subgroup of men are predisposed to fatal heart disease at an early age.[28]

Do women on estrogen therapy have less heart disease? No one seems to have a definitive answer. For every study to show a protective benefit of estrogen, there is another that shows an increased risk of heart disease among users, or no difference at all.[29]

Proponents of estrogen therapy point to the fact that estrogen creates a healthier HDL-LDL balance, and seems to reduce clogged arteries in women who have had total hysterectomies. But the following evidence cannot be ignored:

• Men with existing heart disease who received a daily dose of estrogen were seen, in one study, to be twice as likely to die from a subsequent heart attack than men who received a placebo.[30]

• Oral contraceptive pill users have an increased risk of blood clots, heart attacks, high blood pressure and stroke.[31] (It should be noted that contraceptive users are on artificial estrogens in much larger doses than those used to treat menopause.)

• In a small number of women, oral estrogens, even in low doses, can result in an elevation of blood pressure.[32,33] (Blood pressure returns to normal when estrogen therapy is discontinued.[34] And all women on estrogen are advised to have their blood pressures checked frequently by their physicians.)

The increasingly popular use of synthetic progesterones along with estrogen therapy further complicates the heart disease issue. Progestins or progestogens (the synthetic forms of progesterone) may increase the chances of blood clots, strokes and heart disease.[35] What's more, this hormone is thought to upset the favorable HDL-LDL balance that estrogen therapy alone may bring. So progesterone may neutralize any protective heart disease benefits of estrogen.[36]

Cigarette smokers who are thinking about taking estrogen should be aware that smoking and estrogen don't seem to mix very well. Estrogen taken in high doses (much higher than is usually prescribed for menopausal symptoms) can alter blood-clotting patterns and cause thrombophlebitis (inflammation of a vein with formation of blood clots). Smoking somehow alters the body's chemistry so that even small amounts of estrogen can dangerously alter blood-clotting patterns.[37]

To summarize, there is no conclusive evidence—pro or

con—about estrogen therapy and heart disease. The studies that do exist don't clearly distinguish between estrogen users and those on a combination estrogen/progesterone regimen, or between women who have surgical menopause and those who have a naturally occurring menopause. Only initially healthy women, without a history of heart disease, are selected to go on estrogen therapy; and this further biases study results.[38] In the meantime, women with past or present cardiovascular disease are advised not to go on hormone therapy.

Other Research Findings

While estrogen therapy is relatively safe when taken with the proper precautions and follow-up care, the following research findings have been noted in the literature:[39,40]

1. Women taking estrogen are two to three times more likely to have gallstones requiring surgery than are non-estrogen users.

2. Estrogen can increase fibroids and endometriosis, conditions that would normally clear up by themselves if no hormone therapy were taken.

3. Estrogen and progestogens increase fluid retention, so that conditions affected by this must be carefully watched (e.g., asthma, epilepsy, migraine, and cardiac or kidney disease).

4. High levels of estrogen may cause benign liver tumors and may alter blood sugar metabolism (which is why diabetics need special follow-up care if placed on hormone therapy). Findings on liver tumors and blood sugar levels are based mainly on younger women taking oral contraceptives, and it is uncertain whether or not they apply to the type of low-dose estrogens used for menopausal problems.

Who Should Go on Estrogen Therapy?

In September 1979, approximately 250 physicians, researchers and consumers gathered at the National Institutes of Health to review the facts about estrogen and to make some general recommendations concerning its use. Their consensus was that there is no easy formula for determining who should take estrogen. Every woman must make this decision for herself after weighing the benefits and risks of treatment with her physician. Only the woman herself knows how severe and life-disrupting her symptoms are, or how she feels about possible long-term risks. The conferees did, however, recommend that women use the smallest possible effective dose for the shortest amount of time needed for therapy.[41] These recommendations are still generally followed by most physicians.

Before making any decision about taking estrogen therapy, you'll want to have a long talk with your doctor concerning its benefits, side effects and risks. What type of estrogen does he or she recommend? What kind of follow-up care will you need? Write down on a pad any questions you may have before your appointment. That way you won't kick yourself later because you forgot to ask an important question. And don't be afraid to take notes. You may want to review your physician's comments when you get home. Should you feel uncomfortable with or unsure about one particular physician's approach to treatment, you should never hesitate to seek a second opinion.

During your office visit, your doctor will want to evaluate your health and family history. It is strongly recommended that women do not receive hormone therapy if they have the following conditions: a history of uterine or breast cancer: heart disease; blood-clotting disorders; stroke; and undiagnosed abnormal vaginal bleeding. DES mothers and daughters are also advised against estrogen use.

Physicians have strong reservations about giving estrogen to women with cystic breast disease, high blood pressure, diabetes, liver or gallbladder disease, a strong family history of breast cancer, a history of migraine headaches, and heavy smokers.

Other conditions which may rule out estrogen therapy, or at least involve extremely cautious follow-up care include: fibroid tumors, obesity, epilepsy, asthma, varicose veins and excess blood cholesterol.

Women who expect to have surgery within four weeks are advised not to begin estrogen therapy.[42,43,44]

If you've had an early menopause—either naturally or due to surgery—your doctor will probably recommend that you go on estrogen therapy. An early menopause is associated with a high risk of osteoporosis. (More about this bone-thinning disease will be discussed in Chapter 11.)

If ovaries are removed surgically or destroyed through radiation, a woman is very likely to suffer severe menopausal symptoms, and estrogen is usually recommended. When menopause occurs naturally, severe hot flashes, night sweats and vaginal atrophy are other reasons that hormones might be prescribed.

After assessing your personal history, you should be given a thorough physical examination, including a check of your heart, blood pressure, pelvis, rectum and breasts. A Pap smear and blood and urine analysis should be performed.

Many doctors recommend that an endometrial biopsy be done before you start on hormone therapy, particularly if you are taking estrogen without added progesterone. This procedure can usually be performed in the doctor's office, and involves taking a small sample of the uterine lining for examination. A biopsy can detect cancer or precancerous conditions. (See Chapter 12 for a detailed discussion of this and other office procedures.)

Estrogen Tablets

Most women take estrogen in tablet form. There are two different types of oral estrogens: natural and synthetic. The so-called natural estrogens are made in the laboratory, but come from animal sources. Premarin—the most widely prescribed menopausal estrogen tablet—is derived from the purified urine of pregnant mares. That's how it got its name: Pre (pregnant), mar (mare's), in (urine). Synthetic estrogens are made from artificial, petroleum-type chemicals. They are cheaper to produce and are found mainly in birth control pills. Synthetic estrogens seem to cause more side effects than natural estrogens, especially nausea. But there is no clear evidence as to whether one form of estrogen is safer to use than the other.[45]

Some tablets include a combination of estrogen and tranquilizers. A doctor might prescribe such a combination for a patient who is depressed and anxious. It is important that a patient be informed of the fact that she is taking a tranquilizer. The drug can impair mental and physical functioning, and the ability to perform everyday tasks, such as driving. Long-term use of tranquilizers can be addictive, and a woman can suffer withdrawal effects when she stops the medication. Should there be a medical need for both of these drugs, you are probably better off taking them separately. That way you can taper off the tranquilizer while staying on estrogen, if need be.

Estrogen can also be prescribed in a combination tablet with androgen, or male hormone. The androgen is used as a mood elevator and has been found to improve libido. This combination is used less and less today, as it can cause a woman to develop male characteristics, such as hoarseness, deepening of the voice, excess hair growth and an enlarged clitoris. Some of these changes are irreversible.[46]

A common way to administer estrogen tablets is three weeks on the hormone and one week off. The one week rest period is thought to give the endometrial and breast tissue some rest from the hormone's stimulating effects. During the week off, some women complain that their symptoms return. One woman, who has had a total hysterectomy, describes it this way: "I go twenty-five days on estrogen and five days off. That week off is complete hell for me. My hot flashes come back worse than ever. I feel as if my body is on fire, and am constantly drenched in perspiration. The flashes used to return after I was off estrogen for a day. But my doctor upped the dosage and now the flashes don't start happening until the third day."

Researchers in Sweden are experimenting with the uninterrupted use of estrogen and progesterone with some success.[47] Another alternative approach is to give estrogen from Monday to Friday only.[48] The majority of physicians, however, prefer to give estrogen in a cyclical fashion in the belief that this is the best way to help reduce cancer risks.

The usual dosage range for estrogen tablets is between 0.3 to 0.625 mg. (or its equivalent). Doses may be adjusted upward or downward, depending on a woman's reaction to the drug. In addition to Premarin, other common commercial brands of estrogen include: Estinyl, Menest, Evex, Ogen and Estrovis.

Vaginal Creams

Vaginal creams may be prescribed for women who complain of severe vaginal dryness. (Other measures for relief of vaginal dryness are discussed in Chapter 9.) Estrogen cream is applied vaginally, with a tamponlike applicator. Scientists used to think that the creams were safer than tablets and that they affected only the vaginal lining. However, vaginal creams are now known to be absorbed more quickly into the bloodstream than are oral tablets. So if you were to take the same amount of estrogen vaginally as by mouth you would have a much higher concentration of estrogen in your blood.[49]

Estrogen creams have the same risks and benefits as oral estrogens. They will clear up hot flashes and night sweats along with vaginal atrophy.

Most women begin by using vaginal creams once nightly for the first week and then two or three times a week—or as needed thereafter. As the vaginal walls respond to the estrogen they become thicker, and estrogen is absorbed through the vagina at a lowered rate.[50]

You need a far smaller amount of estrogen vaginally than you do orally. Sometimes just a fraction of the applicator amount appears to be effective. "I can tell when I need to apply some cream, just by the way it feels when I'm walking," says one estrogen cream user. "I'll use just a smidge three or four times a week, and it seems to work."

The exact minimum effective dose of estrogen is still a source of medical study.

Adding Progesterone to the Therapy

Doctors in increasing numbers are prescribing synthetic progesterone along with estrogen to ensure the shedding of the uterine lining and to guard against endometrial cancer. Progestin tablets are taken along with the estrogen tablets, usually during the last ten to fourteen days of treatment. Some doctors recommend progestins even for patients who have had a hysterectomy. They feel that it might have a protective effect against breast cancer. However, this view is not shared by all doctors.

When synthetic progesterone is added to estrogen therapy, women commonly experience vaginal bleeding during the drug-free week. This withdrawal bleeding occurs most often during the early menopausal years. Ninety-seven percent of women will experience the bleeding until age sixty. By age sixty-five, only 60 percent will be bothered by it.[51] The bleeding is shorter and scantier than a normal period, usually lasting no more than two or three days each month. Some women find it a nuisance. But it is a necessary way to shed the extra cells that have built up on the uterine lining.

Progestins are now given in lower doses than they used to be, and physicians are still in the process of evaluating the ideal dosages and length of administration.

Other Ways to Take Estrogen

During the reproductive years estrogen is produced mainly in the ovaries and passes directly into your bloodstream. When a woman takes an estrogen tablet, the hormone travels via a different route. It must first pass through the liver before it reaches the blood. There it is broken down into a weaker form of estrogen.

Perhaps half of the estrogen taken orally actually reaches the bloodstream.[52] A large amount remains concentrated in the liver where it may cause changes in liver function and aggravate existing liver problems. It may also affect blood clotting and blood pressure factors.

Some physicians feel that it would be more desirable to bypass the liver and give estrogen in a more direct manner. Alternate ways of giving estrogen are being tested, as follows:

Injections

Estrogen may be injected under the skin in doses that last from three to six weeks. A woman taking estrogen in this way would have to keep returning to her doctor for repeated injections. In addition, the therapy can't be immediately discontinued once injected. This could pose a problem if any complications arose.

Implants

Implant pellets are small, compressed time-release tablets containing a natural estrogen. They release the hormone slowly into the bloodstream for anywhere from three to six months. The pellet is placed into the fatty tissue above the pubic hairline, or in the buttocks or lower back. The entire implant procedure takes five minutes and can be done using a local anesthetic in the doctor's office. Implant pellets would end the daily nuisance of taking pills. However, as with injections, they cannot be removed in the event of side effects or complications. This method has been used in France and the United Kingdom and is being tested clinically in studies in the U.S.

Topical Application

Estrogen cream, when placed directly on the skin, is absorbed directly into the bloodstream. The skin acts as a reservoir and continues to deliver estrogen into the blood for one to two days after it is applied. Researchers at the Center for Climacteric Studies in Florida are testing out the use of skin patches that deliver very small amounts of estrogen to the blood in a continuous and controlled manner.[53] When the skin patch is removed, they find that estrogen levels quickly fall; so the dose and length of treatment is easy to control.

Vaginal Ring

A ring containing estrogen is placed in the vagina where it releases the hormone at a constant rate for weeks or months. The ring is easy to insert and remove and may be left in place during intercourse. It can be left in place for three weeks and then removed for one week, much as estrogen tablets are administered. This method was developed in 1979 and is still in an experimental stage.[54] Some experts feel it may cause an excessive buildup of cells in the vaginal walls.[55] Much more testing needs to be done before it could be made available for general use.

Sublingual Wafers

A wafer containing estrogen is placed under the tongue where it melts into the skin. While much of the estrogen is absorbed directly into the bloodstream, considerable amounts may still pass through to the liver.[56,57] So this method does not totally avoid all of the pitfalls of oral estrogens.

Oral estrogen tablets still remain the method of choice for most physicians. They are painless and easy for a woman to take, and it is easy to increase or decrease the dosage as needed, or to stop treatment altogether. Still, these other methods offer hope for women who are unable to tolerate oral estrogen.

Length of Treatment

How long should a woman stay on estrogen? That depends upon the reasons she is taking it. Hot flashes and night sweats usually require short-term treatment, lasting anywhere from six months to two or three years.

Estrogen does not cure hot flashes. It only postpones them. The aim of therapy is to help a woman's body to gradually adjust to lower hormone levels. The initial doses of estrogen may be relatively high, to bring prompt relief, but are then gradually tapered off.

When a woman goes off estrogen therapy cold turkey, she is likely to have flashes as bad, if not worse, than they were before. Doctors usually wean women off estrogen very gradually, allowing their bodies ample time to adjust. This weaning process may last from two to three months.[58]

The treatment of vaginal atrophy and osteoporosis, on the other hand, may require many years of therapy. When estrogen creams or tablets are discontinued, vaginal dryness may return and bone loss accelerates. Since long-term treatment with hormones is involved, the usual practice is to administer the lowest possible doses.

There are some doctors who still maintain that estrogen should be used by all women—whether they have symptoms or not—from menopause to grave. This philosophy, however, is not shared by the U.S. Federal Drug Administration, the

World Health Organization, or the American Medical Association's Council on Scientific Affairs, all of whom recommend the lowest possible doses of estrogen for the shortest period of time necessary for therapy.[59,60,61] In their package inserts, manufacturers of estrogen also warn against the possible risks of long-term estrogen use.

Possible Side Effects

As with any drug, estrogen may have side effects. Not everyone experiences them. But while you are undergoing treatment you should be on the alert for any unusual body changes and report them at once to your doctor. The following are some of the side effects that have been reported among estrogen users.

Abnormal Vaginal Bleeding

Vaginal bleeding is a common side effect of estrogen. However, any abnormal spotting or bleeding must be reported to the doctor at once, as it can be an early warning sign of uterine cancer. The scanty bleeding that occurs during the drug-free week among women on estrogen-progesterone combination therapy is considered normal, and not a cause for concern. However, even scheduled withdrawal bleeding, if much heavier or more prolonged than usual, requires medical follow-up.

Abnormal vaginal bleeding usually calls for an endometrial biopsy or a D & C. Should hyperplasia be discovered, it often clears up by itself when therapy is stopped, or if progesterone is added, or given for longer periods of time.

B₆ Deficiency

As with oral contraceptives, there's evidence that estrogen therapy may result in a vitamin B_6 deficiency. The symptoms of this are increased depression, emotional instability, fatigue, inability to concentrate, insomnia and loss of libido. The addition of a vitamin B_6 supplement seems to easily solve this problem.[62]

Nausea

Approximately 20 percent of all estrogen users complain of nausea during the first two or three months of therapy. In many cases the nausea goes away by itself after three or four weeks, and all that is necessary is an antiemetic medicine. One physician suggests that taking tablets with the evening meal may be helpful.[63] Sometimes the estrogen dosage has to be decreased.

Excess Fluid Retention

Estrogen users sometimes note that their breasts become engorged and tender, and that they put on extra weight. There may be bloating and pelvic discomfort due to swelling tissues. "My breasts and nipples felt so sore that they hurt when I brushed my hand against them," says one woman. Sometimes reducing the estrogen dose, or using a different hormone preparation, helps to relieve this problem. Some doctors recommend diuretics, while others caution against their use. Water retention seems to become less severe by itself over time.

Headaches

Some women experience severe headaches on estrogen. "It's like a vise is screwed on my head. No amount of aspirin helps. I have to go right to bed." If the problem persists, the doctor may advise you to stop therapy.

Estrogen therapy is not recommended for migraine sufferers. Migraines seem to naturally disappear in about 75 percent of women after menopause. Hormone treatment may prolong these attacks, and may even make them worse in severity and duration.[64]

Other Side Effects

Other possible problems resulting from estrogen use include increased cervical mucous secretion; elevated blood pressure; alterations in coagulation, fat and blood sugar profiles; skin discoloration; and a worsening of fibroids and endometriosis. A change in the curvature of the cornea may make contact lenses impossible to wear.

Side Effects of Progesterone

With the addition of progesterone, some women develop premenstrual symptoms, and may not feel as well during the days that they are on this drug. Other possible side effects of progesterone are breakthrough bleeding, bloating, irritability, tension, headache, changes in libido, weight increase or decrease, nervousness, insomnia, edema, jaundice, lack of scalp hair, itching, rashes, growth of excess hair and erythyma (too many red blood cells).

Follow-Up Care

Should you decide to go on estrogen therapy, it's important that you understand the need for regular, ongoing medical screening. Your general health must constantly be monitored, and dosages of the hormones adjusted when necessary.

Your doctor will probably want to see you again a few months after you start therapy to make sure that you are not having any problems with the treatment. After that you will probably be seen every six months or at least annually.

An annual endometrial biopsy is usually performed on women who are taking estrogen only. However, those on estrogen-progesterone therapy may also be advised to have a biopsy after being on therapy for a few years.

At each visit you should have a pelvic and breast exam, and your blood pressure should be checked. In addition, you should be performing your own monthly breast self-examination at home. (See Chapter 12 for more details.)

Report any unusual discomfort, pain or symptoms to your physician immediately. Possible danger signs to look out for are: abnormal vaginal bleeding or spotting; pain in calves or chest; sudden shortness of breath; severe headaches; unusual lumps or swellings; jaundice; dizziness; vision changes; and yellowing of the skin or eyes.

Benefits Vs. Risks

There is no doubt about it. The decision to go on estrogen therapy is a complicated one. There are no easy rules to follow. And every woman must make the decision based upon her own personal situation.

When deciding whether or not to take hormone treatment you have to weigh the benefits of that treatment against the possible risks. It might be helpful to ask yourself the following questions: How severe are your symptoms? Is relief of these symptoms worth the return of monthly vaginal bleeding, the need for annual endometrial biopsies, or the increased chance (though small with good follow-up care) of endometrial cancer and other possible side effects? Do you feel comfortable with the idea of being on medication, or are you the type to worry yourself sick over every possible long-term health consequence?

The FDA makes it mandatory that drug manufacturers provide a patient leaflet outlining the possible risks and side effects of estrogen and progesterone. Ask your druggist for these package inserts. You may want to read these leaflets carefully before making up your mind.

Consider exploring nonhormonal alternatives to relieve menopausal symptoms. Suggestions on diet, exercise and relaxation techniques are mentioned throughout this book.

If you do decide you need estrogen therapy, make sure that you receive continuing medical follow-up care and that you adhere carefully to dosage instructions. Stay alert to possible side effects, and report them promptly to your physician.

Try to keep abreast of the latest developments in hormone therapy. The field is a growing one, and changes occur rapidly. Inform your physician of any new information that concerns you. Says one woman: "I'm always photocopying articles on new information I come across, and sending them to my doctor. My physician and I have a good back-and-forth relationship. I've sometimes pointed out to him new things that he wasn't yet aware of."

Reevaluate your need for continued therapy at each doctor's visit. The goal should be to stay on therapy at the lowest dose for the shortest time possible.

Estrogen therapy can be of tremendous value in cases where women are suffering from severe menopausal symptoms. It appears to be relatively safe if taken with the proper precautions and follow-up medical care.

Chapter 7
Eating
Right

Medical experts are now documenting what mother always knew: that eating wisely promotes good health. Diet is thought to play a major role in the development of a host of diseases, among them cancer, heart disease, diabetes, high blood pressure and osteoporosis, the bone-thinning crippler that strikes 25 percent of women after menopause.

Good eating has added advantages for you as you pass through menopause. At times of stress your body needs extra nutrients to fight illness. And menopause—with its extreme physical and emotional changes—is certainly a time when you ought to bolster your nutritional arsenal.

During your middle years your body is changing, and for a number of reasons your eating patterns have to change as well. For one thing, people usually become less physically active as they age, and therefore burn up fewer calories each day. To add to that, your metabolism is slowing down. It is estimated that you need from 2 to 5 percent fewer calories to maintain your weight every decade after the age of twenty. By your fortieth birthday you may have to cut at least one hundred calories a day from your diet to stay the same weight.

After menopause, you no longer require energy to keep your reproductive system going at full swing, and so your daily calorie needs decline even further. A woman past menopause may have to cut her calorie intake by an additional 10 to 15 percent in order to maintain her weight. (Of course, all of these figures will vary somewhat depending upon your individual lifestyle, metabolism and activity level.)[1,2,3]

Unfortunately, the body's ability to absorb vitamins and minerals from the foods we eat becomes less efficient as we age. So you are hit with a double whammy: you need to cut back on calories to maintain your weight, and at the same time increase your nutritional intake in order to remain in good health. The foods you select must be low in calories, yet packed with essential nutrients.

How to Eat Right

There are fifty nutrients that we know to be essential to the functioning of the human body. They are chemical substances that come from our food as it is being digested. These nutrients cannot be produced by our bodies, or at least not in large enough amounts to meet our needs. They are classified into six groups: protein, carbohydrates, fats, vitamins, minerals and water. These nutrients supply energy, build and repair the body's tissues and regulate body processes.

You don't have to be a dietitian, or pore over detailed nutrition charts to make sure that you are getting the proper nutrients. But you do have to eat a wide variety of foods of different colors and textures from the four food groups. These include:

The Meat Group

Meat (beef, veal, pork, lamb), fish and shellfish; poultry; eggs; legumes such as dry beans, peas, lentils and peanuts; and nuts. The meat group supplies protein, niacin, iron and thiamin (B_1). Two servings a day are recommended. (A serv-

Declining Calorie Needs

The number of calories needed to maintain your weight decreases as you age. The following demonstrates the average daily needs of a 120-pound woman at different life stages.

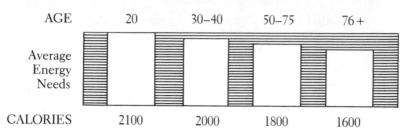

AGE	20	30–40	50–75	76+
Average Energy Needs				
CALORIES	2100	2000	1800	1600

Source: The statistics were adapted from Recommended Daily Allowances, *National Academy of Sciences, Washington, D.C. 1980.*

ing can be 2 ounces of lean meat, fish or poultry; two eggs; 1 cup of cooked dry beans, peas or lentils; 4 tablespoons of peanut butter; or 1/2 cup of cottage cheese.)

The Fruit and Vegetable Group

Includes all fresh, canned, frozen and dried fruits and vegetables, except dried beans and peas. (Dried beans and peas are classified in the meat group since they have significant amounts of protein.) This group supplies vitamins A and C. Four daily servings should include a citrus fruit or juice. (A serving is equal to 1 cup of raw fruit or vegetable, 1/2 cup cooked fruit or vegetable; 1 medium piece of fresh fruit; or 1/2 cup of juice.)

The Milk Group

Milk, cheese, yogurt, ice cream and any milk-containing foods, such as puddings and creamed soups. The milk group supplies calcium, protein and riboflavin (B_2). The recommended requirement is two servings daily; however, some experts believe that women over forty need four servings from this group a day. (One serving equals 1 cup of milk; 1 cup of yogurt; 1 1/2 slices or 1 1/2 ounces of cheese; 2 cups of cottage cheese; or 1 3/4 cups ice cream.)

The Grain Group

All grains such as barley, buckwheat, corn, oats, rice, rye and wheat and the bread, cereals and pasta products made from them. Supplies carbohydrates, thiamin (B_1), iron and niacin. Four servings daily are recommended. (One serving is equivalent to a slice of bread; 1 cup of cold cereal; 1/2 cup cooked cereal, pasta, rice, cornmeal or grits; or 5 saltine crackers.)

Others

Butter, cream, oil, dressings, spreads, candies, cakes, cookies and empty calorie junk foods. These items provide few nutrients and should be eaten sparingly.

Special Needs at Menopause

Are there any special nutritional requirements for a woman of menopausal age? Scientists are just beginning to address themselves to this question. While special Recommended Daily Allowances have been set for infants, children and women who are pregnant or lactating, there are none for the woman who is going through menopause. Nutrition charts lump adult women into two age groups—twenty-three to fifty and fifty to seventy-five—without special regard to the climacteric years. Only lately is it being realized that the menopausal woman may have some unique needs of her own.

One major example is the Recommended Daily Allowance for calcium set forth by the Federal Drug Administration. According to nutrition charts, women aged fifty-one to seventy-five need 800 mg. of calcium daily. Many medical authorities think this figure is too low. At menopause, women tend to lose calcium from their bones at an accelerated rate. For some this leads to osteoporosis, a condition in which the bones become thin and easily fractured. An adequate amount of calcium in the diet is believed to help prevent this disease. It may also offer protection from high blood pressure and help the body to cope with stress. Experts are now advising that women over forty consume from 1,000 to 1,500 mg. of calcium daily. That's the amount of calcium in four glasses of milk or its equivalent.

In our calorie-conscious society, many women cut down on milk products beginning in their teens. "I haven't had milk with my meals since I was a kid," confides one woman. "I usually drink coffee or a diet soda instead. I wouldn't want to squander all of my calories on a glass of milk." A survey conducted in 1977–78 revealed that 42 percent of the population, especially females over eleven and males over thirty-five, consumed less than 70 percent of the Recommended Daily Allowance for calcium.[4]

If you have been negligent about including calcium in your diet, you may want to gradually increase the amount you consume. Milk and dairy products are, by far, the best sources. Choose products made from skimmed or lowfat milk rather than whole milk—they're healthier for you and easier on the waistline. Get into the habit of drinking milk with meals, or as an in-between-meal snack. If you don't like drinking milk, you can sneak it into creamed soups (instead of water), or add nonfat dry milk to stews and casseroles. Have yogurt for lunch. Custards, puddings and ice cream are milk-containing desserts. Or healthier yet, top off your meal with cheese and fruit.

There are many good nondairy sources of calcium in the diet too. These include dark green leafy vegetables (collards, turnip greens, spinach, broccoli), salmon and sardines with their bones, oysters and calcium-containing tofu. You can also try adding a small amount of vinegar when cooking meat bones for stews and soups. The vinegar dissolves the bone and produces a calcium-rich broth. The table on page 125 will give you some idea of the relative amounts of calcium in different foods.

Though you may be getting enough calcium, your body will not be able to properly absorb it unless you consume sufficient amounts of vitamin D. Vitamin D is called the sunshine vitamin, because our bodies can manufacture it when our skin is exposed to the sun. You need at least fifteen minutes to an hour of exposure to the sunlight each day to satisfy your body's need for vitamin D.[5] However, pollution, inclement weather, lifestyles and work habits often conspire to deprive us of our daily sunshine quota. And we have to look to the foods we eat to take up the slack.

Milk sold in this country is fortified with vitamin D and is the best source of this nutrient. Vitamin D is also available in cod liver oil, egg yolk, saltwater fish and liver. The ability to manufacture vitamin D decreases as we age, and some experts think that the Recommended Daily Allowance of this nutrient should be raised for older women.[6]

Some things in your diet can interfere with your body's ability to absorb calcium. When a person's diet is overloaded with too much protein, for example, she may lose calcium from her bones in increased amounts. Soft drinks contain high levels of the mineral phosphorous, which hampers calcium absorption. So can an excess of dietary fiber, and certain medications such as aluminum-containing antacids, laxatives, cortisone, tetracycline, thyroid preparations and diuretics. Excessive amounts of smoking, alcohol, caffeine and salt can all upset your body's calcium balance.[7,8]

Calcium Supplements

Some people simply can't tolerate milk. It gives them cramps, gas, bloating and diarrhea. They have what is known as a milk sugar or lactose intolerance. The degree of sensitivity to lactose varies. Some people can digest small amounts of milk with their meals, or can eat cheeses and yogurt with no problem. Others have digestive problems from even the smallest traces of lactose. There are special milk products available in supermarkets and health food stores which should be helpful in such cases. These include acidophilus and soy milks, as well as milks that are specially processed to break down the offending milk sugar. There is also a product on the market known as Lact-Aid, an enzyme which helps to make milk more digestible. Four to five drops are added to a quart twenty-four hours before you drink it. (It breaks down the milk sugar and gives the milk a sweet taste.) Lact-Aid can be purchased in health food stores, pharmacies and some supermarkets. Or you can write to the address at the back of this book.

If you are among those who cannot tolerate milk, or you just don't like it, you may want to consider taking a daily calcium supplement. Beware of dolomite and bone meal, both of which have been used as calcium supplements. They are

What Foods Contain Calcium?

Food	Calcium
Milk Products	
Whole milk, 1 cup	291 mg.
Lowfat milk, 1 cup (2 percent)	297 mg.
Skim milk, 1 cup	302 mg.
Buttermilk, 1 cup	285 mg.
Lowfat yogurt, 1 cup (plain)	415 mg.
Lowfat yogurt, 1 cup (fruit-flavored)	345 mg.
Brick cheese, 1 oz.	191 mg.
Cheddar cheese, 1 oz.	204 mg.
Cottage cheese, 1 cup (2 percent, lowfat)	154 mg.
Swiss cheese, 1 oz.	272 mg.
Ice cream or ice milk, 1 cup	176 mg.
Meat Group	
Beans, dried, cooked, 1 cup	90 mg.
Oysters, raw, 7 to 9	113 mg.
Shrimp, canned, 3 oz.	90 mg.
Pink salmon, with bones, 3 oz. (canned)	167 mg.
Sardines, with bones, 3 oz. (canned)	372 mg.
Tofu, processed with calcium sulfate, 4 oz.	145 mg.
Vegetables (Fresh, Cooked)	
Bok choy, 1 cup	252 mg.
Broccoli, 1 cup	136 mg.
Collards, 1 cup	358 mg.
Kale, 1 cup	206 mg.
Mustard greens, 1 cup	194 mg.
Spinach, 1 cup	167 mg.
Turnip greens, 1 cup	252 mg.

Sources: *USDA Handbook Nos. 8-1 and 456, and* The All American Guide to Calcium-Rich Foods, *National Dairy Council, 1984.*

potentially toxic and best avoided. Dolomite comes from rock material made up mainly of calcium and magnesium. But some samples have been found to contain toxic minerals such as lead, arsenic, mercury and cadmium. Bone meal, too, may be contaminated with these and other toxic metals.

Calcium carbonate or calcium lactate are the most used and least expensive calcium supplements. Calcium gluconate may also be prescribed, but is more expensive. These supplements most commonly come in tablet form, but may also be prescribed in powders or liquids. "Chelated" calcium tablets, sold in many health food stores, claim to enhance calcium absorption. They are very expensive. And there is no medical proof that they are any better than other calcium supplements.[9]

It doesn't seem to matter which form of calcium you use— all appear to be absorbed equally well. However, each supplement contains a different percentage of calcium. And this affects the price of the product as well as the number of pills you have to take per day. Calcium carbonate contains the highest amount of calcium (40 percent), while lesser amounts are found in calcium lactate (13 percent) and calcium gluconate (9 percent).[10] This means that you'd have to chew far fewer calcium carbonate tablets a day to reach your desired total.

Several over-the-counter antacid tablets are made entirely of calcium carbonate, flavoring and sweeteners—the same ingredients as in some other, more expensive commercial tablets—and may be used as calcium supplements. Tums and Alka II, for example, contain 200 mg. of calcium per tablet. Read labels carefully, however. Antacids containing aluminum, such as Maalox, Mylanta, Gelusil and Riopan, can actually interfere with calcium absorption.[11]

Calcium carbonate may cause gas and constipation, but some manufacturers add magnesium to the formula, and that usually takes care of this problem. Your physician may also want to give you a vitamin D supplement to make sure that calcium is properly absorbed. However, most healthy people get enough of this vitamin from sunshine and the foods they eat. Since vitamin D is toxic in high amounts, never take supplements without your physician's approval.

It is generally recommended that you spread out your supplements over the course of the day, retaining about one third of the dose for bedtime (your body loses more calcium during sleep).[12] Those with a history of kidney stones should consult their physician before taking calcium supplements, and everyone taking supplemental calcium should drink adequate liquids each day. This keeps urine volume up, and decreases the possibility of kidney stone formation.

When calculating how many calcium tablets you need, take into consideration the amount of calcium that you usually consume through foods. The supplements should fill the gaps left by your diet. (For a discussion on specific recommended dosages, and the question of possible calcium overdosing, see Chapter 11.)

Vitamin Supplements

If you are eating a nutrient-rich diet with a variety of choices from each of the four food groups, you probably don't need to take vitamin supplements. A sensible, well-rounded diet will take care of all of your nutritional needs.

There are times, however, when vitamin supplements may be necessary. If you've failed to take proper care of yourself during pregnancy and lactation, for example, you may reach your middle years nutritionally depleted. Or your body may temporarily require extra nutrients during times of extreme emotional stress, illness or surgery. Perhaps you are dieting and sacrificing valuable nutrients along with calories. Often women who live alone don't take the trouble to prepare well-balanced meals for themselves. Says one woman, who was recently widowed: "Why bother making stews or casseroles just for yourself? Usually I'll come home from work and grab a peanut butter sandwich or a can of soup for dinner." In cases such as these, a multivitamin pill that supplies you with the adult minimum daily requirements may be taken as a form of insurance, but it should not be considered a substitute for nutritious foods.

Vitamins have become big business in this country. Many people take them in megadoses, feeling that if a little is good, a lot must be better. This is dangerous reasoning. Certain vitamins, in excess, can be hazardous to your health. This is especially true of oil-soluble vitamins, such as A, D, E and K, which are stored in the body for long periods of time.

Consume too much vitamin A, for example, and you may end up with hair loss, cracked lips, dry skin, severe headaches, general weakness, blurred vision, a susceptibility to bruising and nose bleeds, painful joints, emotional disturbances, fatigue and insomnia. Go overboard on vitamin D and you may experience nausea, weight loss, weakness, excessive urination, diarrhea, depression, irritability, hypertension, calcification of soft tissues, including blood vessels and kidneys, bone deformities and multiple fractures.

Vitamin E is stored in the body in very small amounts, and is less toxic than either vitamin A or D. But even this vitamin, in high doses, can have negative consequences. Some people find too much vitamin E makes food become less appetizing. High amounts of this vitamin have been known to cause weight gain, blurred vision, blood clots, indigestion, high blood pressure, skin rashes and sleepiness.

People don't normally take supplements of Vitamin K, which helps the blood to clot, unless they have some serious illness or are on certain medications. Vitamin K in excess can result in vomiting and dangerous blood clots.

Water-soluble vitamins are less toxic than oil-soluble vitamins. They are not stored for very long within the body. And excess amounts are excreted in the urine. Yet even water-soluble vitamins can pose health problems if taken in excessive amounts. Too much vitamin C, for example, may result in diarrhea, cramps, kidney stones and kidney damage, excess urination and abdominal pain.[13,14]

A nutrition educator for the National Dairy Council sums it up this way: "Vitamins in megadoses, even water-soluble vitamins, can do more harm than good. Vitamins and minerals interact with one another in highly complex ways. Too much or too little of one can affect the body's absorption of another. The issue is confusing and complicated. And there are a lot of doctors out there who aren't really knowledgeable about the good or bad effects of these nutrients."

The best source of advice on nutrition, she says, is a registered dietitian: "If you have any questions about your diet,

What Vitamins Do for You

Vitamins	Functions	Best Sources
A	Healthy skin, eyes and mucous membranes. Helps eyes adapt to dim light. Increases resistance to infection.	Dark green leafy and yellow vegetables, yellow fruits (e.g., carrots, sweet potatoes, chard, spinach, turnip greens, apricots), liver, fish liver oil, fortified milk.
B complex	For good digestion and a healthy nervous system. Promotes healthy skin, particularly around the mouth, nose and eyes. Helps the body utilize fats, carbohydrates and protein.	Whole grains, brewer's yeast, lean meats, organ meats, poultry, fish, dried beans and peas.
C	Keeps skin supple and elastic. Hastens healing of wounds and bones. Increases resistance to infection. Aids in utilization of iron.	Citrus fruits and juices, broccoli, strawberries, cantaloupe, tomatoes, cabbage, green peppers, potatoes, green leafy vegetables, sprouts.
D	Helps the body to use calcium and phosphorous, necessary for strong bones and teeth. Important for heart action and nervous-system maintenance.	Fish-liver oils, egg yolk, fortified milk and milk products, organ meats, fish.

What Vitamins Do for You (Continued)

Vitamins	Functions	Best Sources
E	An antioxidant (prevents deterioration of tissues due to action of oxygen). Protects red blood cells and fat-soluble vitamins. Thought by some to help alleviate hot flashes.	Wheat germ, whole grains, vegetable oils, eggs, green vegetables, beans, peas, seeds, nuts, organ meats.
K	Important for blood clotting.	Green leafy vegetables, fruit, dairy products, whole grains.

you might want to contact a dietitian on staff at a nearby hospital, or phone your local dietitian's association."

Treating Menopause with Nutrition

Some women say certain nutritional supplements have helped to alleviate their hot flashes and other menopausal symptoms. Beneficial claims have been made for calcium, vitamins B, C, and E and bioflavonoids. (See Chapter 3, Hot Flashes, for a more complete discussion.) Vitamin B_6 has been used with reported success to alleviate tension, fatigue and depression, and to reduce water retention and swelling. (However, some women find that vitamin B_6 makes them nauseated and dizzy.)[15]

While these nutritional supplements may be helpful, it cannot be stressed enough that they should be taken only under professional supervision. As we indicated earlier, all supplements have the potential for being toxic in large amounts.

It can't hurt to add these nutrients to your diet in the form of wholesome, nutritionally rich foods. If you feel depressed or irritable, think about sprucing up your diet with foods rich in B vitamins. Sprinkle a handful of wheat germ on your salad or in stews or casseroles; mix some brewer's yeast into your morning juice, or toss it on unsalted popcorn for a snack (use nutritional brewer's yeast, the sweet-tasting kind). Concentrate on eating whole grains and whole grain breads and cereals rather than refined or processed products. Calcium is good for relief of tension, as well as for keeping your bones strong. So you might want to drink extra milk or snack on dairy products during times when you feel especially stressed.

Relaxation techniques can also help to enhance your feeling of well-being. You may want to review the ones that have been outlined for you in Chapter 5, Getting "Up" and Out. Regular exercise, too, can be a natural mood elevator and relaxant.

Foods to Avoid

It's common for women to experience exaggerated premenstrual symptoms as they move through their thirties and forties. The accumulation of several extra pounds of water in the week or so before your period can cause breast tenderness, swelling, weight gain, headaches, irritability and insomnia. Some women feel better if they cut down or eliminate caffeine, alcohol and sweets from their diets. (If you're a heavy coffee drinker, you'll want to cut back on caffeine very gradually, perhaps by one to two cups a day. Caffeine withdrawal can cause such symptoms as headache, drowsiness, nervousness, depression and even nausea and vomiting. These symptoms may occur within twelve to sixteen hours after the last dose.) It may also be helpful to limit your salt intake for a week to ten days before you expect to menstruate.

Salt does more than just aggravate premenstrual bloating. Excessive amounts of it may contribute to high blood pressure and to the loss of calcium, a mineral which women in their menopausal years can ill afford to be short on. And in countries such as Japan, Iceland and China, where the main food staple consists of pickled and salt-cured foods, the rates of cancer of the stomach and esophagus are high.[16,17]

The ingredient in salt that may pose a problem is sodium. Sodium is vital to our bodies' functioning. It helps to regulate blood volume and pressure, and to transmit nerve impulses. But many people grab for the shaker and sprinkle generously despite the fact that they already get more than enough sodium in the foods they normally eat. Animal products, such as meat, fish, poultry, eggs and milk are naturally very high in sodium. Fruits and vegetables have sodium too, though in lesser amounts. Sodium is also a prime ingredient in baking soda, baking powder, MSG, emulsifiers, canned and cured foods, processed foods, soy sauce, relishes, catsup, mustard and flavor enhancers.

The average American consumes 4,000 to 4,500 mg. of sodium each day (there are 2,000 mg. of sodium in a teaspoon of salt). That's several times the amount we need, providing we are not performing some strenuous physical chore on a sweltering summer day. Because approximately one third of this sodium intake comes directly from the salt shaker, either during cooking or at meals, a logical place to cut back on salt would be in our own kitchens.[18,19]

Spare the kitchen salt, and wake up your tastebuds. Salt masks the natural taste of foods. And once you get used to doing with less of it, you will begin to appreciate those hidden flavors. Try using lemon juice and different herbs and spices as substitutes for salt. Garlic and onion powder and pepper are good stand-ins (but garlic and onion *salts* are simply salt with added spices). Open your spice jars and experiment with new taste sensations. You might want to prepare this salt-substitute mixture, published in the April 1984 issue of *FDA Consumer* : Mix in a blender 2 teaspoons of garlic powder and 1 teaspoon each of basil, oregano, powdered lemon rind (or dehydrated lemon juice). The resulting mixture should be stored in a glass container to which rice is added to prevent caking.[20] There are lots of innovative ways to use spices, and many standard cookbooks have charts with helpful suggestions.

Diuretics

If your water retention problem is especially severe, your doctor may recommend that you take a diuretic, or water pill, in addition to reducing your salt intake. Diuretics have a tendency to deplete the body of its potassium supply and can result in weakness, fatigue and leg cramps. So most physicians counsel users to eat foods high in potassium each day. These include bananas, cantaloupe, honeydew, nectarines, raisins, grapefruit juice, potatoes and avocados. Sometimes a potassium supplement is prescribed along with the diuretic.

Diuretics may also result in zinc depletion if used for prolonged periods of time. Signs of zinc depletion are a decrease in the sense of smell and taste, impairment of night vision, a decreased ability of wounds to heal and, in men, impotence.[21]

Never take diuretics without medical supervision. They can cause dehydration and possible heart rhythm abnormalities.

Smoking and Alcohol

No one can dispute the fact that smoking is detrimental to your health. Cigarette smoking is responsible for 30 percent of all cancer deaths, and smokers have a ten times greater chance of developing cancer than nonsmokers. Smoking has been linked to the development of heart disease; chronic bronchitis; emphysema; cancer of the throat, lung, mouth, pancreas and bladder; and to minor respiratory infections and stomach ulcers.[22,23] Just being near other smokers, and inhaling the air in a smoke-filled room can be harmful to your health if the exposure is long-term.

Smoking, in some as yet unknown way, can lead to an earlier menopause, and may increase your risk for developing osteoporosis and endometrial cancer. Women who smoke heavily appear to have more bone fractures in later life, especially if they are slender and are not on estrogen therapy.[24] Research indicates that female smokers with osteoporosis may be three times more likely to lose their teeth than nonsmokers.[25]

But the good news is this: once smokers quit, the negative effects of cigarette smoke seem to reverse themselves rather dramatically. The health risks of ex-smokers seem to be closer to those who never smoked than to those who refuse to kick the habit.[26]

Smoking doesn't mix well with alcohol either. The combination of the two in excess leads to a higher incidence of cancers of the mouth, throat and larynx.[27] (Anything over one to two drinks per day is considered excessive.) Alcohol is high in calories, and robs the body of vitamins and minerals that are vital to a woman in her middle years, including calcium and the B vitamins. It is associated with cirrhosis, liver cancer, brain damage and obesity.[28] All good reasons *not* to drink to your health.

Dietary Fiber

As the body ages, and the metabolism slows down, you may find that your digestive system is a bit more sluggish too. Constipation may become an annoying problem. It is not a good idea to get hooked on laxatives as a long-term solution. Laxatives rob the body of essential nutrients, and also create a dependency, so that your bowels can no longer function on their own. Stool softeners are more gentle than laxatives. But better yet is the use of fibrous foods in your daily diet.

In grandma's day fiber was known as roughage. It is the indigestible portion of the plants we eat. Fiber acts like a sponge, absorbing several times its weight in water so that the stool becomes bulkier and passes more quickly through the intestines. That means less straining and pressure on the bowels and surrounding blood vessels.

Americans used to eat a lot more fiber a generation ago. But our diets have become high in sugars, fats and processed foods. Some scientists think that this is why Americans and citizens of other industrialized nations have a high incidence of colon cancer while populations eating high-fiber diets do not.[29] Fiber is believed to dilute cancer-causing substances in the bowel. And by speeding the passage of waste matter, it is thought to reduce the amount of time that the intestine is exposed to cancer-causing agents. (Other scientists blame high colon cancer rates on excessive fats in the American diet.)[30,31]

Fiber has other health advantages too. It may relieve hemorrhoids (varicose veins of the rectum). And it is believed to help prevent diverticular disease, which an estimated 40 percent of all middle-aged Americans suffer from.[32] (Diverticulitis involves the formation of pockets in the intestinal lining which may become painfully inflamed or infected.) Fibrous foods are low in calories but give a feeling of fullness, which makes them a plus in any weight control diet. However, easy does it when adding fiber to your diet. If you are not used to eating a lot of fiber, you may, in the first weeks, feel gassy and bloated. A gradual change in diet may eliminate these possible discomforts

Foods high in fiber include whole grains, and whole grain products, such as breads and cereals; fresh fruits and vegetables, especially when eaten with the skins, peels and pulp, and beans, peas and seeds. (Prune juice, though not high in fiber, also has a natural laxative effect.) Some manufacturers add wood pulp to breads, baked goods and ice cream. This is not the same as the dietary fiber in fresh foods, and not enough is known about the long-term effects of ingesting wood pulp.[33]

To increase the amount of fiber in your diet, you might try tossing barley, brown rice or beans into soups and casseroles. Add bran, sunflower seeds or chopped fruit with the peels on to yogurt and cottage cheese. Or eat raw, unpeeled fruit as a snack. Cooked potatoes should be eaten with their jackets, and applesauce or baked apples with their skins. Avoid loading up on just one type of fibrous food. There are at least six different types of fiber, and each has advantages unique to it. And don't be overzealous about fiber either. Excessive amounts may interfere with the absorption of calcium, zinc, iron, magnesium, phosphorous, copper and vitamin B_{12}.[34]

If constipation is a problem for you, you'll also want to be sure to drink plenty of liquids each day (at least six to eight glasses), and to exercise regularly. Regardless of whether or not you have the urge, try to establish a regular time for elimination. Never postpone going to the bathroom when you feel the urge to do so, and don't hurry yourself once you're there.

Fats and Cholesterol

Americans may be dying of affluence. Too much fat and cholesterol in our diets may make us targets for heart disease and various types of cancer. We consume four times the amount of fat that inhabitants of less industrialized nations of Asia, Africa, and Central and South America do. In fact 40 percent or more of the American diet consists of fat.[35,36]

A moderate amount of fat in our diet is necessary. Fat promotes growth and healthy skin. It provides concentrated energy and cushioning for vital body organs. Fats transport the fat-soluble vitamins A, D, E and K through the body.

There are different kinds of fats. Polyunsaturated fats (usually a liquid oil from a plant source) are thought to help lower cholesterol levels in the blood and reduce chances of heart disease. Saturated fats (solid at room temperature, and derived from animal sources) are thought to build up on the inside of arterial walls and contribute to hardening of the arteries, stroke and heart attacks.

In the interest of preventing heart disease, since 1961 the American Heart Association has recommended a low-saturated-fat, low-cholesterol diet. However, more recent reports indicate that all types of fat may contribute to tumor development. So, in 1982, the National Academy of Sciences Committee on Diet, Nutrition and Cancer recommended that *total* fat consumption (of both saturated and unsaturated fats) be reduced to 30 percent of the American diet.

Although it hasn't been conclusively proven, the link between high-fat diets and cancer has been observed in studies of large populations. One 1975 study, for example, showed a direct correlation between death rates from breast cancer and per capita fat intake in thirty-nine countries. The Japanese, who eat a traditionally lowfat, high-fiber diet, have low rates of breast and colon cancer. But they begin to develop these cancers after they migrate to the United States and adopt American eating patterns.[37] Groups of people within the U.S. who eat lowfat diets, like the Seventh Day Adventists, have lower rates of breast and colon cancer than the rest of the population.[38]

Studies of laboratory animals also show a link between fats and cancer. Animals fed diets high in fat were more likely to develop cancer of the breast and colon. Lean and underfed animals developed fewer tumors than their overfed counterparts.[39,40]

Consider the following suggestions to reduce the fat level in your diet:

• Limit your use of oils, gravies, butter, cream, lard and fatty meats. These are the foods that are highest in fat.

• Choose lean meats, fish, poultry, dry beans and peas as protein sources (The American Heart Association recommends no more than 6 ounces of lean meat, fish or poultry a day. One cup of vegetable proteins—dried beans, peas, legumes—is equivalent to 2 to 3 ounces of meat, yet has only traces of fat.)

• Bake, broil, boil, stew or roast meats instead of frying them. Skin fat off poultry before cooking, and trim all traces of fat off meats before preparing.

• Use lowfat dairy products rather than whole milk.

• Moderate your consumption of egg yolks, organ meats and shellfish, all high sources of cholesterol. Whole eggs (the most concentrated source of cholesterol) should be limited to no more than three a week, according to the American Heart Association.

• When following a recipe, use less oil or butter than called for, and use two egg whites in place of one whole egg. If preparing omelets you might toss out every other yolk.

Red meats and egg yolk have gained a bad reputation because they add fat and cholesterol to the diet. But they happen to be good sources of iron, too. So while it may be healthy to cut down on these foods, be cautious about cutting them out entirely. Over-vigilance can result in anemia.

If you must cook with fat, choose liquid vegetable oils and margarines, which are rich in polyunsaturated fats, over butter and other solid cooking fats. Learn to read food labels carefully for the amounts and types of fats that foods contain.

If a margarine lists "liquid vegetable oil" as its main ingredient, it is high in polyunsaturated fat. If the label reads "hydrogenated vegetable oil" or "partially hydrogenated vegetable oil," then it has less polyunsaturated fat. Coconut and palm oils, though in liquid form, are saturated fats and should be avoided.

Summary

It is not easy to change a lifetime of eating habits. But if you want to look and feel good and stay healthy as you age, it is essential. What nutrition experts advise boils down to the following:

1. Eat a varied, well-balanced diet from the four food groups.

2. If you're over forty, step up the calcium in your diet.

3. Go easy on salt, refined sugars and empty-calorie junk food, especially if you are experiencing exaggerated premenstrual symptoms.

4. Cut down on caffeine intake.

5. Eat luncheon meats (sausage, baloney, etc.) and salted, smoked or cured meats sparingly.

6. Drink alcohol only in moderation.

7. Stop smoking.

8. Increase foods that are high in fiber.

9. Cut down on fats.

A change in diet can add excitement to a menu grown bland with familiarity. One woman, who recently started adding whole grains, lentils and beans to her family's usual meat-and-potato diet, says that she finds the exploration of new foods to have perked up her interest in cooking again: "I love going through the bins of the health food department, discovering new tastes and new ways of cooking. I've begun taking home some of the more exotic vegetables that I've never cooked before and replacing some of our main meat meals with vegetarian casseroles. I'm having fun shaking up our old eating habits and putting some surprises on the table." With the right attitude healthy eating can be a pleasurable change rather than a bothersome chore.

Chapter 8
Exercise:
The Best
Anti-Aging
Pill

Ours is a push-button, drive-through world. The marvels of technology have brought us cars, elevators and self-powered electrical appliances—all of which take the muscle out of daily living. For relaxation we curl up in front of a TV, popcorn bowl and remote control switch in hand. The result of this mixed blessing? By the time we reach our middle years, our untaxed bodies function less efficiently: hearts weaken, arteries clog up, digestive systems become sluggish and muscles turn to flab.

Many of the things we attribute to menopause and aging are really due to disuse. Physical exercise, says the National Institutes of Health, is the "most effective antiaging pill ever discovered."[1] It does more to keep you trim, limber and feeling good than anything else. Agrees one physical education specialist: "People who don't exercise have less energy, flexibility, strength and endurance. The body, after all, is like a machine. If it is not used over a long period of time, it will not run smoothly. Joints become rusty, your range of motion limited, and you put on pounds. By failing to exercise, you are really doing yourself harm."

Do Your Health a Favor

Vigorous exercise pays extra dividends after menopause, when the incidence of heart disease among women increases. It is an excellent all around conditioner for your cardiovascular system. Regular physical activity keeps your heart stronger and pumping more efficiently. And it raises the level of HDLs, the blood proteins that help keep arteries clear of fatty deposits. Your lungs, too, reap benefits. They expand and contract more fully and take in more oxygen per heartbeat. Exercise can reduce high blood pressure. And, by and large, it reduces a person's risk of developing hardening of the arteries, stroke and heart attack.[2,3]

By exercising regularly, you'll boost your spirits along with your pulse rate. Vigorous activity acts as a natural mood elevator and relaxant. In fact, researchers have found regular exercise to be more effective than drugs in treating patients with mild to moderate depression.[4,5] Exactly why exercise has this mood enhancing property is unclear. But there are several possible explanations.

First, and most simply, exercise provides a welcome reprieve from daily stresses. As one avid swimmer describes it: "When I'm in the pool doing my laps it's as if I'm on a minivacation. My husband, the kids, my job—all of that seems far away. It's just me and the rhythm of my body chugging through the water. I'm in my own little world." Says another woman, recently widowed, "My exercise classes give me something to look forward to each week. They get me up and out of the house and among other people. It's better than sitting home feeling sorry for myself."

Exercise can cause changes in the chemistry of your brain. People who jog, for example, secrete more endorphins, a morphinelike substance that deadens pain and creates a feeling of well-being.[6,7] This naturally produced chemical is responsible for the runner's "high" and for feelings of nervousness and irritability among runners when they miss a day or two of exercise.

As you exercise, the flow of oxygen to your brain increases. And this, too, may account for an improved sense of well-being. So may the fact that exercise promotes deeper, more refreshing sleep. People who stick to a regular exercise program also enjoy positive feelings of accomplishment and control over their lives.

You reduce your risk of developing osteoporosis when you exercise, especially if you are getting plenty of calcium besides. People who are bedridden for prolonged periods experience severe and rapid bone loss. But those who regularly perform weight-bearing exercises (the kind that put stress on your bones) develop stronger, denser bones than their sedentary counterparts.[8] (More about this in Chapter 11.)

You'll look a lot better too. Physical activity turns excess body fat to muscle, and helps to curb middle-age spread. It also burns up more calories—an especially welcome bonus when you consider that your need for calories declines after menopause.

There are several more pluses to add to the exercise scorecard: it's good for digestion; helps speed the process of elimination; prevents stiffening of arthritic joints; aids in the control of diabetes; and keeps coordination and reflex responses sharp well into old age.

Inactivity breeds boredom and fatigue. But exercise can energize you. As the experts note, there is no guarantee that exercise will add years to your life, but it will certainly add life to your years.

Before You Begin

If you have led a fairly sedentary life up until now, you'll want to take certain precautions before embarking on any strenuous exercise program. Start by consulting your physician. He or she will probably want to give you a complete physical examination to make sure that you're in good health. According to the American Heart Association, you should also consult a physician if you have any of the following conditions:[9]

• Heart trouble, a heart murmur or a previous heart attack.
• If you have high blood pressure that is not under control, or you don't know whether or not your blood pressure is normal.
• You have frequent pressure or pain in the chest, neck, shoulder or arm after exercise.
• You experience breathlessness after mild exertion.
• You have bone or joint problems.
• You often feel faint or have spells of severe dizziness.
• You have a medical condition that needs special medical attention (for example, insulin-dependent diabetes).

Sometimes an exercise stress test, performed by a physician, is in order. The stress test can often spot potential heart problems. Some doctors routinely perform one for people forty and over, or for anyone who is considered at risk for heart disease (for example, heavy smokers; those with high blood pressure, elevated cholesterol levels, diabetes, or a family history of heart attacks; and severely overweight individuals).

Stress tests are commonly conducted in the doctor's office or in a hospital laboratory. They usually take about fifteen minutes, during which time you are placed on a treadmill and attached by electrodes to an electrocardiogram machine (ECG). The treadmill is gradually tilted and its speed increased so that you end by walking rather briskly up a slight incline. During the stress test, changes in your heart rate are recorded on the electrocardiogram and your blood pressure is constantly monitored. Any abnormal dips in the ECG or sharp fluctuations in blood pressure may be possible warning signs, as may pain that develops in the chest, or spreads into the neck, throat, shoulder or left arm.

Getting Started

Anything worthwhile takes work and perseverance. And so it is with exercise. It may take at least six weeks to get your body into shape. And at first you'll need considerable resolve to shake those old sedentary habits.

You might find it helpful to find an exercise "buddy"—your spouse or a friend—so that you can help spur each other on. One sixty-four-year-old woman relates how she and her neighbor began a walking regimen that has continued daily over the past fifteen years:

"Margie and I used to meet in the mornings and kibitz over coffee. Instead of stuffing our mouths with donuts, one day we decided to start the day off with a morning walk. Through the years several other women have joined us, and a bunch of us meet at six A.M. every morning throughout the year. We walk quite briskly, for about five miles. Not even subfreezing temperatures or snow can hold us back. I've made many lovely friends this way. And I get to feast my eyes on some truly stupendous sunrises."

If you don't have a partner, and need some guidance and moral support, check out your local YMCA, YWCA or community center. There are many types of ongoing exercise classes, and at most facilities there are trained professionals who would be happy to help you select an appropriate exercise program.

Aerobic Exercises

To *really* exercise your heart and lungs, you need to perform an aerobic exercise. Aerobic means, literally, "of air." It is the type of activity that speeds your heart rate, increases your breathing and pumps more oxygen to every part of your body. Walking, running, hiking, swimming, aerobic dancing, bicycling and cross-country skiing all fall into this category.

Anaerobic forms of exercise do not require as much oxygen. They may build muscles, but they won't do as much for your all-around physical conditioning. Weight lifting is an example of an anaerobic exercise.

Be prepared to devote a minimum of thirty minutes, three times a week to exercise. Research has shown that you need at least this amount in order to stay in optimal shape. (Ten of these minutes should be devoted to warming up and cooling down, and twenty minutes to continuous aerobic activity.)

Five exercise sessions a week would be even better, if you can spare the time.[10]

Pick an aerobic activity that you find pleasurable and that you'll want to make a permanent part of your lifestyle. The following is a brief rundown of some common aerobic exercises. There's no reason why you can't combine several of these activities into your overall exercise plan.

Walking

Walking is probably the best activity for an exercise novice. It takes no athletic skill. It's easy on the joints. And everyone knows how to do it. If done properly (at a brisk, arm-swinging rate that brings your heart rate up) it is an excellent cardiovascular conditioner. You can burn up the same number of calories by walking one mile as you can by running the same distance. The only difference is, walking takes more time. Walking does little to build the upper body. And you may want to supplement it with another sport or exercise that does.

Jogging

A superb cardiovascular conditioner. But it takes time and patience to build up to it, especially if you've been sedentary. (See "Exercise Guidelines," on p. 147.) Like walking, jogging does little to develop your upper body. Some runners carry weights, or perform another sport or exercise.

Swimming

Nearly the perfect exercise, swimming builds cardiovascular fitness and develops all major muscles in the body— including legs, arms, back and stomach. It doesn't put stress on bones, joints and muscles, which makes it ideal for the elderly and for anyone with joint problems, but a drawback in terms of keeping bones strong. If you enjoy swimming you should alternate it with a program of walking, bicycling or some other weight-bearing exercise that will help to reduce your chances of osteoporosis.

Bicycling

A good cardiovascular conditioner that requires little athletic prowess. It is somewhat better than walking and jogging for upper body development, particularly if the handlebars are dropped style.

Aerobic Dance

Great for those who enjoy moving their bodies to the beat of popular music. It combines the fun of dancing and the benefits of aerobic exercise. Stretching movements and dance routines impart flexibility and strengthen both upper and lower parts of the body.

Cross-Country Skiing

This is an excellent aerobic sport. As it is seasonal, it should be part of a steady, year-round exercise plan.

Racquetball/Squash/Handball

These activities provide cardiovascular conditioning only if the ball can be kept in play for sustained periods. They may be a bit too strenuous for the beginning exerciser.

Tennis

Expert singles players who maintain long, fast rallies may stay fit through tennis. But the game involves too much stop-and-go activity to provide good aerobic conditioning for most people. Supplement with a regular program of aerobic exercise.

Jumping Rope

Should be done only if you are already in top-notch physical condition, as it accelerates the heart rate very quickly. You may want to skip five minutes and walk in place five minutes until you build up to more.

Ice Skating/Roller Skating

Good aerobic conditioners only if you're very proficient at them, and can sustain the activity at a steady pace for twenty to thirty minutes.

What to Wear

Comfort, not style, is what counts when you're dressing to exercise. If you're walking or jogging, it pays to splurge on a first-rate pair of running shoes. Look for thick, flexible soles that will absorb the shock when your feet hit the ground. Adequate cushioning can help prevent damage to the bones and ligaments in your feet, ankles, knees and hips. Make sure that the shoe gives you good arch support. And allow half a thumbnail of space at the toe. Any reputable sports supply store should be able to assist you in making the proper selection.

Exercise clothing should be loose-fitting and made of material that allows your skin to "breathe." A good supporting cotton sports bra will add to your comfort, especially if you are large-breasted.

Don't overdress, no matter what the season. You don't want sweat-soaked clothes against your skin. In warm weather, cotton T-shirts and shorts are sensible choices. Light colors will help to deflect the sun's rays, and on hot, sunny days a white cotton hat can help to keep you cool.

You can be comfortable when properly dressed even on the coldest of winter days. Dressing in layers is the secret. Layers prevent the cold and wind from penetrating to your skin. And they can be peeled off or added again as necessary. The layer closest to your skin should be made of cotton, as it helps to keep your body dry. On really frigid days make sure that your head and extremities are well protected. Wear a wool hat or ski mask, warm wool socks, and warm gloves or mittens. A turtleneck will help to keep your neck warm without the bulk of a scarf.

Some people exercise in rubberized sweat suits, thinking that if they perspire a lot, they'll lose more weight. This is both false and dangerous. The weight lost from perspiration is replaced just as soon as you drink more water. By dehydrating yourself you run the risk of heat exhaustion or heat stroke.

For safety's sake, wear bright colored or fluorescent clothing at dawn or dusk. Walk or run while facing oncoming traffic, and stick as close as possible to the shoulder of the road. Try to exercise where the traffic flow is not too heavy. But avoid running in isolated areas alone.

Bicyclists should get into the habit of wearing a safety helmet whenever they ride. Keep long pants secured with a bicycle clip; and use fluorescent tape or reflectors on pedals and wheels, as well as on the front and rear of the bike. Avoid cycling in inclement weather and when visibility is poor; and ride with the flow of traffic, obeying all traffic rules and sticking close to the shoulder of the road.

When swimming, choose a lightweight bathing suit that hugs your body in a streamlined fashion. Make sure that the shoulder straps are sturdy, and that the suit doesn't bind you anywhere. A good pair of swim goggles is a must for serious lap swimmers, especially when the water is highly chlorinated.

If you're exercising solo, there's an optional purchase that can take the boredom out of your exercise routine: a portable radio or cassette player with earphones, which will allow you to exercise to the accompaniment of music, talk shows or even to a crash course in a foreign language. There are all sorts of lightweight radios and cassette players on the market that have been designed with the exerciser in mind. They're great to use in the park, on an indoor track or on a fitness trail or stationary bike. Be cautious about using earphones in traffic, though. It's important that you remain alert to the sounds of oncoming vehicles.

Exercise Guidelines

Exercise should be an enjoyable, safe and satisfying part of your life. To keep it that way:

1. *Start slowly and build up gradually.* Enthusiastic beginners often plunge headlong into exercise, trying to do everything at once, but slow and steady are the keys to a program of lifelong fitness. Says one physical education instructor: "When people set out on an exercise program they often overdo it—swimming, running and bicycle riding all on the same day. Then they burn out quickly, and give the whole thing up. Be reasonable in setting your exercise goals. If you don't start gradually you'll end by being terribly sore, or even injuring yourself. You'll quickly be discouraged and won't rush back to try it again."

Gradually increase the intensity and duration of exercise. If you're out of shape, ten minutes of brisk walking may be plenty for you at first. Add several additional minutes each week, and before you know it, you'll be able to walk twenty, thirty or even forty minutes at a clip.

If you've never jogged before, you might want to get into condition by walking briskly the first few weeks. Begin each subsequent session with a brisk walk, and then alternately walk and jog, gradually building up to the point where you are jogging the entire time.

The same rule of thumb applies to swimmers. Begin by doing as many laps as you can without undue strain, and slowly increase thereafter. Most swimmers find the breast stroke to be less demanding than the crawl, and you may want to alternate between the two.

2. *Exercise at a safe target heart rate.* Aerobic exercise should not be so vigorous that it overtaxes you, or so inefficient that it fails to adequately raise your pulse. You should be striving to reach 60 to 70 percent of your maximum pulse rate. This is known as your target heart rate. To calculate your target heart rate subtract your age from 220, and multiply by .60 or .70, depending upon how advanced you are in an exercise program. A forty-year-old woman just starting to exercise would find her target heart rate as follows:

$$220 - 40 = 180 \text{ (Maximal pulse rate)}$$
$$180 \times .60 = 108 \text{ (Target heart rate)}$$

To determine whether or not you are exercising within your target heart rate, take your pulse immediately after you stop exercising. For this you'll need a stopwatch or a wristwatch that measures time in seconds. Find your pulse by lightly pressing the first two fingertips on the thumb side of your wrist or over one of the blood vessels on your throat, just below the angle of your jaw. Your pulse can also be felt by placing the first three fingers on your temple. Time the number of pulse beats that occur over a ten-second period, being sure to count the first beat as zero. Then multiply the number of beats by six. (It's a good idea to practice pulse-taking in a nonexercise situation until you become adept at it.)

If your pulse falls somewhere below your target heart range, you'll want to put a little more oomph into your exercising. If it falls above, take it a little easier. Take your pulse at least weekly over the first few months of exercising, and then periodically thereafter.

You can pretty much tell for yourself when you are overdoing it. When you exercise within the proper range you should not become so breathless that you cannot manage to carry on a conversation or to sing aloud. You can very gradually increase your target heart rate over the months, going to 65 percent (multiplying your maximal pulse rate by .65) and then to 70 percent (multiplying your m.p.r. by .70) as your body becomes better conditioned. If you are in the very pink of condition and have been exercising for at least six months you may even exercise at 85 percent (multiplying your m.p.r. by .85) of your target heart rate, according to the American Heart Association, however, it is not necessary to exercise that hard in order to stay in good physical condition.[11]

3. *Don't neglect to warm up and cool down.* Each and every exercise session should begin with a warming-up period lasting five minutes. Warm-ups give your heart and muscles a chance to gradually adjust to increasing levels of activity. They bring an increased blood flow to muscles and surrounding tissue, and help to prevent injuries to muscles, ligaments and joints during exercise. Properly warmed-up muscles are less likely to ache after exercise.

At least five minutes of cooling-down exercises are also necessary to help your body wind down to a resting state. When you stop exercising abruptly, blood tends to pool in your legs. Blood pressure may take a dip, causing you to feel lightheaded or possibly faint. In extreme cases, a heart attack may occur. A more gradual decrease in exercise assures that your leg muscles will continue to contract and keep the blood circulating back to your heart.

Warm up and cool down by stretching the muscles you are about to use, and then performing a low-level version of your chosen activity. Walkers and runners should concentrate on limbering their leg muscles. (See suggested stretches on the next page.) Swimmers, who use all major body muscles, should do overall body stretches, involving legs, arms, shoulders and waist.

A stretch should be a gentle form of exercise, without any fast bouncing movements. Each stretch should be held about

Suggested Stretches for Warming Up and Cooling Down

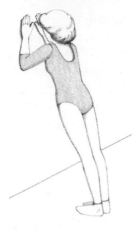

WALL PUSH

1. Stand 1½ feet away from the wall.
2. Lean forward and push your palms against the wall at eye level (heels remain flat on the floor).
3. Hold for 15 seconds.

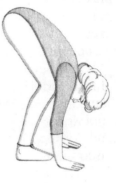

PALM TOUCH

1. Bend knees slightly.
2. Try to touch the floor (without bouncing) by bending from the waist.
3. Hold for 15 seconds.

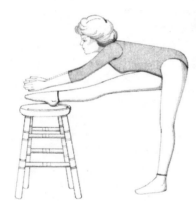

TOE TOUCH

1. Place your right leg on a chair, stool, or railing, so that the knee is straight and leg parallel to the floor.
2. Keep your left leg straight and lean forward, reaching for your toes.
3. Hold for 15 seconds (don't bounce).
4. Repeat with opposite leg.

fifteen to thirty seconds, until a slight discomfort is felt, and then released slowly. Repeat each stretching movement two or three times. Remember to continue breathing in a normal, relaxed way throughout.

After the muscles are limbered, you'll want to ease into an increased activity level. Walk briskly for several minutes before jogging and then gradually accelerate to your accustomed pace. If bicycling, pedal leisurely on flat ground at first (on a stationary bike, set the resistance lower for the first and last five minutes). A swimmer might want to do a few flutter kicks on the side of the pool, and then take it very easy for the first two laps. After twenty or thirty minutes of vigorous exercise, you should gradually decelerate your activity level and cap off the exercise session with another round of stretch exercises.

4. *Heed warning signs.* Your body will tell you when you are pushing it too hard. Listen to it. Stop exercising if you feel nauseous, dizzy or extremely fatigued, and if you find that you have difficulty breathing. Severe cramps, a pale complexion and pain in the chest, or anywhere else, are also signals to cease activity. You should be pleasantly tired after an exercise session, but not wiped out for the entire day. In fact, it's common to feel invigorated about an hour after exercising.

If you have not exercised in many years, or are using groups of muscles that you do not normally exercise, be prepared for some muscle soreness in the early weeks. Proper warm-up and cool-down exercises should help to minimize this problem, and heating pads and warm baths will ease the temporary discomfort.

5. *Drink plenty of fluids.* Always keep your body well hydrated, drinking liquids both before and after you exercise. This is especially important in hot, humid weather. If the air is saturated with moisture, perspiration cannot evaporate and cool the body as it should. The result can be heat exhaustion, a condition characterized by fatigue, nausea, listlessness, confusion and faintness.

Should you experience symptoms of heat exhaustion, stop exercising at once and drink plenty of fluids. Failure to do so can result in heat stroke, a more serious condition that requires medical attention.

To guard against heat exhaustion, don't exercise as long or as intensely when the thermometer soars above 82 degrees or the humidity rises above 60 percent. Exercise when the sun's rays are weakest—either in the early morning or late afternoon. And pick a walking or running route that offers shady cover. On days of extremely high humidity, you'd be wise to postpone exercise altogether. Be sure to drink lots of water before and after physical activity. And on very hot days, drink small amounts of water during exercise as well.

6. *Make a weekly exercise schedule and stick to it.* Don't

squeeze exercise into your life in a haphazard fashion, or you're likely to chuck it at the first excuse. Your health is one of your most important priorities. Is thirty minutes out of a sixteen-hour waking day really too much to devote to it? You may well find, as one woman does, that the self-discipline required for exercise spills over into other areas of your life: "When I exercise, I feel more productive and can pack more into my day. But when I skip a few days everything else in my life seems to slide too."

Plan to exercise year-round, no matter what the weather. If you're turned off by the cold, see what indoor facilities are available in your area. Your local parks and recreation department may be able to direct you to indoor swimming pools, running tracks or gymnasiums. Neighborhood colleges and public schools often have indoor sports facilities that are open to the public. And YMCAs, YWCAs and community centers offer fitness classes year-round. You may want to invest in a private health club membership. If you do, visit the facilities first, during the times you would normally be exercising, to see how crowded conditions are.

Some exercisers have found ingenious ways to stick to their regimens: "When it's raining buckets or very cold, my husband and I go to the largest mall in our area," says one retired suburbanite. "We walk from one end clear to the other and back again." Sprawling metropolitan airports offer miles of wide open walking space. Or you might walk briskly through a large museum or department store.

If you're at a loss for a good indoor exercise spot, consider your own living room. You can always turn on some music and dance or run in place. You may want to treat yourself to a stationary bicycle. They don't take up much space, and you can get a really good aerobic workout while parked in front of your TV set, or even while reading a book.

7. *Don't get discouraged.* You can't be an overnight success at exercising, especially if you've been neglecting your body for decades. But you are sure to notice some measurable results by the six- to ten-week mark. You will be less easily winded for one, and able to exercise for longer periods without feeling fatigued.

You might want to keep an exercise diary to record your progress. At each session, write down your exercise heart rate, the distance or amount of time you exercised, and how you felt afterward (e.g., "breathless," "tired," "exhilarated"). That way you'll have tangible evidence of your accomplishments. Set some attainable short-term goals for yourself, too, like swimming two extra laps in the pool by week's end. Then hand yourself a mental trophy. You deserve to feel proud.

8. *Don't rest on your laurels.* Exercise benefits cannot be squirreled away like money in the bank. You must constantly exercise to maintain your cardiovascular health. It takes a mere two to three weeks of inactivity to lose all of the exercise benefits you've worked so hard to accrue.

Exercise, Diet and Weight Control

The fat in our bodies is a form of energy insurance. In more primitive times it provided a reserve of calories for emergencies, when food supplies were scarce. Today, most of us can—and do—walk to our refrigerators whenever the mood strikes. The fat stores in our bodies accumulate to an unhealthy level. The result: over half of all Americans are overweight.[12]

Each pound of excess body fat represents 3,500 calories of unused energy. If you want to shed some of this extra fat, you have two choices: eat less food or burn more calories. By eating 500 calories less per day, you can lose one pound of fat a week. If you burned up an additional 500 calories a day through physical activity, you'd lose two pounds weekly. This combination—of cutting calories and stepping up exercise—is far better than either approach alone.

The 200 to 300 calories burned in thirty minutes of exercise don't seem as if they'd make a dent in terms of weight loss. But the effects of exercise are cumulative. Just a small increase in physical activity can result in weight loss over time. If you were to take a half-hour walk after dinner each day, you would be five pounds lighter at year's end. If you jogged three miles, five times a week, you'd drop two pounds a month, or a total of twenty-four pounds a year.

When you diet, you lose weight from lean muscle tissue as well as from fat stores. Your scale may tip in the desired direction, but your body will still look flabby. Exercise burns off excess fatty tissue while building up lean muscle mass. It helps to firm your body as you lose weight and keeps you feeling healthier.

You'd think that exercising would increase your appetite. On the contrary, moderate activity seems to keep a lid on overeating. When given a daily dose of exercise, laboratory animals will eat less than their sedentary counterparts.[13]

Exercise speeds up your metabolism, and keeps it raised for up to six hours after the activity. So you burn extra calories both during exercise and afterward. That's several additional pounds of fat lost a year—without any special effort on your part.

There is some evidence that you can burn more calories when you exercise several hours after eating than you do on an empty stomach.[14] You might want to capitalize on this by planning your exercise sessions accordingly.

Obesity: Hazardous to Your Health

Your need for calories may decline with each passing decade, but your ideal weight remains what it was at twenty-five. (See ideal weight chart on the next page.) The amount of calories you as an individual need per day depends upon your age, height, activity level and metabolism. A very active woman can eat a few hundred calories more than one who is sedentary. And a large-framed woman will burn more calories during physical activity than one who is small-boned. Roughly speaking, a woman past menopause needs about fifteen calories per pound to maintain her weight.[15]

How much weight is too much? Anyone 20 percent over her ideal weight is considered obese. Obesity has been linked to many major health problems, including high blood pressure, hardening of the arteries, diabetes, gallbladder disease, hernia, arthritis, heart disease and certain cancers. In 1985, a National Institutes of Health panel called obesity "a killer" in the same sense that smoking is. Even an extra five or ten

What You Should Weigh

The following are normal weights for American women between twenty-five and fifty-nine years of age. Heights are in feet and inches (assuming shoes with 1-inch heels) and weights are in pounds (assuming indoor clothing weighing three pounds).

Height	Weight (small frame)	Weight (medium frame)	Weight (large frame)
Women			
4–10	102–111	109–121	118–131
4–11	103–113	111–123	120–134
5–0	104–115	113–126	122–137
5–1	106–118	115–129	125–140
5–2	108–121	118–132	128–143
5–3	111–124	121–136	131–147
5–4	114–127	124–138	134–151
5–5	117–130	127–141	137–155
5–6	120–133	130–144	140–159
5–7	123–136	133–147	143–163
5–8	126–139	136–150	146–167
5–9	129–142	139–153	149–170
5–10	132–145	142–156	152–173
5–11	135–148	145–159	156–176
6–0	138–151	148–162	158–179

Source: 1983 Metropolitan Life Insurance Company height and weight tables.

pounds can be hazardous to your health, this panel of experts cautioned.[16]

It's more difficult to keep your weight in check as you grow older. A slowing metabolism and a decrease in physical activity conspire to help you put on the pounds. If you are eating the same way as you did at twenty, and are exercising less, it's a good bet that you've got a battle with the bulge on your hands.

A *Thin Lifestyle*

Americans seem to have an unrequited love affair with dieting. Books that promise instant weight loss rise to the top of best-seller lists, and diet aids have become a multimillion-dollar industry. But all of this frenzied dieting seems an exercise in futility: about 95 percent of dieters regain their lost weight within a year.[17] As one perennial dieter jokes: "It's easy to lose ten or fifteen pounds in a few weeks. I've done it hundreds of times."

Gimmicky diets usually concentrate on one type of food. There are high-protein diets, high-carbohydrate diets, and diets in which you eat grapefruits, bananas or some other single food ad nauseum. A calorie is a calorie, no matter what food it comes from. And the success of these diets is due to the monotony of the menu—not to any magical properties of the food. Most fad diets are nutritionally unbalanced, and can jeopardize your health. They are not a long-term solution to a chronic weight problem. If they were, why would so many new diets crop up each year?

If you really want to lose weight and keep it off, you have to change your lifestyle for good: exercise regularly; cut down on fried, fatty foods and empty-calorie junk foods; eat smaller portions of nutritionally rich foods from the four basic food groups (see Chapter 7).

Before you begin an exercise and diet plan, you should consult your physician, particularly if you have any special health problems. Buy yourself a calorie counter so that you can keep an accurate record of how many calories you are consuming each day. And consult the exercise chart on the next page to get an idea of the amount of calories you can burn off during a regular weekly exercise schedule.

A weight loss of one to two pounds per week is a goal that's sensible and realistic. Just increase your physical activity and decrease your food intake to the point where you use up 500 to 1,000 calories more per day. You can lose weight on a varied, nutritionally balanced diet that satisfies all of your health requirements. If you restrict your diet to below 1,200 calories a day, however, you'll need to take supplemental vitamins and minerals.[18]

Calories Burned During Twenty Minutes of Activity

Activity	Calories Used
Easy walking	60
Golf (flat course)	90
Brisk walking	100
Gymnastics	140
Heavy gardening	140
Dancing	160
Tennis	160
Skiing (downhill)	160
Skiing (cross-country)	180
Rowing	180
Racquetball or handball	200
Brisk jogging	210
Bicycling	220
Swimming	240

Source: American Medical Association, "Personal Health Care," Newsweek supplement, Oct. 29, 1984.

Some find it helpful to join a dieter's support program. Weight Watchers, Overeaters Anonymous and TOPS (Take Off Pounds Sensibly) are three groups that adhere to nutritious, sensible dieting plans and help members to break poor eating habits.

The following weight loss tips may also be of help:

• *Don't eat unless you feel hungry.* People often eat when they feel bored, lonely, depressed or anxious; or to help them unwind while watching T.V. or reading. Recognize these dieter's pitfalls, and learn to replace habitual nibbling with other behaviors. You could, for example, draw up a list of home projects that you've been meaning to do (needlepointing, reorganizing the family photo album, letter writing, etc.). And when the urge to raid the icebox strikes, attack the tasks at hand instead. If you're feeling nervous or fidgety, take time out for relaxation exercises (see page 75) or go for a long walk.

• *Live an aerobic lifestyle.* Look for ways to add exercise to routine activities throughout your day. Get off the bus a stop before work and walk. Park your car a few extra blocks from your destination. Take stairs instead of elevators whenever possible. You'll keep your cardiovascular system well-conditioned and burn extra calories to boot.

• *Stock your cupboard with low-calorie foods.* Grocery shop with calories in mind. (The best time to cruise the supermarket aisles is when you are *not* hungry.) If you can't resist jelly donuts, don't bring them home. If your family likes ice cream, pick a flavor that doesn't appeal to you. Place all of the tempting "no-nos" in the back of the cupboard or refrigerator where you can't see them. Keep fresh fruit in view, and a big plastic bag of low-calorie munchies handy in the fridge (carrot and celery sticks, green pepper strips, zucchini circles, broccoli spears, etc.).

• *Develop sensible eating habits.* Eat at least three meals a day. Skipping meals can be self-defeating. You'll only be tempted to eat a forbidden snack or to overeat at the next sitting. Try to eat your largest meals early in the day, when you can actively burn off the calories. Ideally, dinner should be the lightest meal of the day.

Don't eat on the run or gobble your food. Instead, sit down, cut your food into small pieces and eat slowly. You're less likely to overeat that way.

To feel really full, eat generous portions of high fiber foods and drink plenty of water during and between meals. Clear soup as an appetizer can help blunt your appetite.

• *Avoid alcoholic beverages.* Alcoholic drinks are high in calories. What's worse, they lower your inhibitions and weaken your willpower. Have a wine spritzer (half wine, half club soda) if you must. Sparkling water with a twist of lemon or lime is a refreshing, calorie-free alternative.

• *Dine out intelligently.* There's no reason for you to forego fine restaurants and social dining just because you're dieting. Order foods that are broiled (with no added butter), poached, baked or boiled. And avoid anything that's fried, sauteed or which comes in a gravy or cream sauce.

Some restaurants will leave sauces or gravies off at your request. And you can ask that salad dressing be brought to you in a separate side dish. That way you can control the amount you put on your salad, and dilute it first with water, lemon juice or vinegar. (You may even enjoy the tang of fresh squeezed lemon juice alone on your salad.) For dessert, ask for fresh fruit or fruit in light syrup.

• *Don't blow your diet.* After losing the first few pounds, you're bound to hit a plateau. It may seem as if your scale won't budge, no matter how diligent your dieting efforts. Don't give up now. If you're eating less and exercising more, it will only be a matter of time until the scale takes another dip.

And if you completely blow your diet, try to hang in there. Don't use this as an excuse to go on an eating binge. Everyone is entitled to an occasional calorie splurge. Just try to compensate for it by eating less or exercising more the following day.

Some physical changes of aging are unavoidable. Tummies grow rounder, waists tend to widen and there is a general redistribution of weight around the middle. If you continue to exercise and watch your calories, you can slow these natural changes and continue to look trim. In most cases, middle-aged spread is just another excuse for overeating and underexercising.

Chapter 9
Sexuality

"Why would sex be worse after menopause? It's better. No more worries!"—Aged sixty-seven.

If sex is an important and enjoyable part of your life it's apt to remain so after menopause. Human sexuality is a lifelong affair. And study after study has revealed that aging adults lead rich and varied sexual lives through their fifties, sixties, seventies and beyond.[1,2,3,4,5]

Sex may be even more pleasurable for you after menopause. Although estrogen levels fall at menopause, your ovaries and adrenal glands continue to produce androgens, or male hormones. Androgens are the sexual "turn on" hormones. Now, unopposed by estrogen, they may exert a more powerful influence on libido than ever before.

From a purely physical standpoint, the capacity for sexual enjoyment increases with age. Sexually experienced women have a larger and more complex network of veins in the genital area, especially after they've borne children.[6] When this venous bed becomes engorged during sexual excitement, it can contribute to heightened feelings of sexual tension.

Practical experience has its advantages too. A mature lover has fewer inhibitions and is more apt to know how to please herself and her partner. She may be liberated from the fear of pregnancy and the nuisance of birth control. And with child-rearing behind her, she finally has the time and privacy to devote to more leisurely lovemaking. It's no wonder so many women compare this phase of their marriage to a "second honeymoon."

"When our youngest son left home for college my husband and I acted like two kids let loose in a toy shop. We romped around the house nude, in the middle of the afternoon, yelling racy things to each other. We feel like young lovers all over again."

In a recent large-scale survey 800 men and women, aged sixty to ninety-one, were found to be as sexually active as forty-year-olds. Did menopause add or detract from their sex lives? Of the 478 women polled, 42.1 percent said that sex was better after menopause; 44.7 percent said there was no change; and 13.2 percent said that it was worse.[7] In other words, the vast majority of women found sex to be the same or better than it was when they were menstruating.

Cultural Myths

Despite all of the evidence to the contrary, our youth-oriented culture tends to view older people as sexual neuters. Sex seems inappropriate or slightly ridiculous among people who are middle-aged or elderly.

"I heard my male colleagues chuckling over one of the patients on the hospital floor. She was sixty years old and had asked the doctor how soon after her operation she could resume sexual relations. From then on she was referred to behind her back as 'the sex lady.'"—A professor of nursing.

It's widely held that as you get older you lose your sexual appetite, function and capability, concurs one sex therapist: "The label 'dirty old man' is commonly used for a sexually active male. As if sex at that age were somehow abnormal or obscene. As for the older woman, we don't even give her the dignity of a sexual epithet. At menopause, society would have you think that she's supposed to take a pause from men.

"As a matter of fact," the therapist continues, "there's another way to look at it. There are many voids in life as you grow older. The parenting function is diminished, so far as caretaking is concerned. Friends die. You may lose your spouse. Retirement can mean that you lose a component of your self-esteem as well. With all of these changes, the need for physical intimacy becomes more of a need, rather than less. If men and women don't fill themselves with self-fulfilling prophesies they are able to be fully sexual throughout their lifetime."

Estrogen and Sexual Desire

After menopause, your body still produces estrogen, but at a much lower rate. Gone are the monthly hormonal peaks and valleys. Hormonal output now occurs at a more steady pace. A logical question to ask is: how does this change in estrogen output affect female sexuality?

The human female is unlike all other mammals regarding her receptivity to sex. Most female mammals go into a period of estrus, or heat, at certain times of the year, during which they ovulate and are most responsive to male advances. The bleeding that occurs during estrus is not the equivalent of a menstrual period. It is, rather, a result of high estrogen levels, much like the spotting that occurs in some women during mid-cycle. When not in heat, most female mammals show no interest in sex.

Sex and reproduction are not one and the same for humans. We hug, kiss, stroke each other and have intercourse to express a deep need to love and be loved. During most sexual encounters women are not even fertile, and having babies may be the furthest thing from their minds. After menopause, when reproduction is no longer possible, the sex urge remains strong.

Many studies have been conducted to see if a woman's sexual desire peaks or wanes at specific times during her menstrual cycle. But there are so many conflicting findings that a consensus cannot be drawn. Several researchers have found that women feel most sexy around the time of ovulation, when estrogen levels are high; and again, just before or during their periods, when estrogen levels are low. Others have found sexual arousal to be greatest after menstruation or in the period before or following ovulation.[8,9,10]

It is clear that there are more things than estrogen at work when it comes to female sexuality. If a woman is in the right frame of mind, she can be receptive to lovemaking at any time during her cycle, whether she is ovulating or not. And she will continue to desire intercourse after menopause, when estrogen levels hit an all-time low.

Your libido is as likely to be affected by your mind as by your hormones. Just as some women discover the joys of sexuality in their menopausal years, and feel liberated from childbearing, others may feel that the loss of fertility desexes them, or that aging makes them less desirable sex partners.

"I'm sagging and flabby, and don't feel very attractive at all. I'm more blasé about sex. It may be fine or not fine. This is upsetting to my husband. He still seems to want me."—Age forty-five.

Common mid-life worries can sap a woman's sexual energies. It's hard to feel sexy when conflicts over elderly parents, adult children or your own life's goals seem to be overwhelming you. Then again, those who never enjoyed sex in the first place may use menopause as an excuse to stop having relations.

Some women experience a temporary loss of libido around the year or two when menopausal symptoms are most intense. Hot flashes and sleepless nights may not be conducive to romance. But as the body adjusts to new hormone levels, sexual interest is likely to return. Says one fifty-five year old: "When my simmering hormones finally settled down, my sex life started simmering."

Estrogen therapy won't help to restore a waning libido. If it does boost a woman's sex drive, it's because it has alleviated severe hot flashes, which can leave a woman exhausted, irritable and unreceptive to sex. Or else it has improved vaginal dryness, a condition which can make sexual intercourse painful.[11,12]

In one study of 502 men and women, ages forty-five to sixty-nine, enjoyment of sexual relations in a person's younger years was the best barometer for determining current interest in sex. Good health and an interested and interesting partner are the other two key ingredients.[13]

Physical Changes

Some physical changes take place in your genitalia and reproductive organs as you age. As estrogen levels fall, your vaginal walls gradually become thinner. The lining loses its characteristic rugations, or ridges, and changes in color from reddish purple to light pink. Both the uterus and cervix shrink in size. And the vaginal secretions become less acidic, which may lead to a higher incidence of vaginitis.

The young vagina is a highly elastic organ that can stretch wide enough to allow a baby's head to pass through it. As you age, your vagina loses much (though not all) of this remarkable elasticity. It becomes shorter and narrower. But it is still perfectly able to accommodate a penis, and does not, in any way, affect your ability to have intercourse.

When a woman first becomes sexually aroused, her vaginal walls secrete slippery droplets that lubricate the vagina, preparing it for penetration. In a young woman this lubrication is copious, and occurs about ten to thirty seconds after she is sexually stimulated. A woman of fifty or sixty may find that it takes from one to five minutes before she notices any wetness. And the amount of lubrication may be less than she used to have.

This combination of shrinking, thinning vaginal walls and decreased lubrication is known in medical terms as vaginal atrophy—a frightening sounding label, and one that's not en-

tirely accurate. Your vagina is not going to wither away with
the passage of time. Indeed, many women are not even aware
of any vaginal changes at all.

Sometimes decreased lubrication will cause some discomfort during intercourse, especially when there isn't enough
foreplay. The nearby urethra and bladder are not as well cush-
ioned because of thinning vaginal walls and may become easily irritated, particularly if sex is prolonged, or if it is repeated
more than once in a short space of time. Some women feel
an urgent need to empty their bladders after intercourse, and
may even feel a burning sensation for two or three days after
having relations.

Vaginal dryness may not become a problem until five or
ten years after menopause. However, the decline in lubrication is not usually a sudden thing. A woman may begin to
notice occasional dryness in her forties, but that it gets progressively worse in her fifties or sixties. Then again, some
women never experience any noticeable changes in lubrication at all. And still others claim that the dryness was bothersome at first, but improved as time went on.

*"I started to have problems with vaginal dryness in my early
forties and went to the doctor. She said that I wasn't aroused
enough. I was very angry at her. It simply wasn't true. We use
KY Jelly to help keep me lubricated. But it's a real pain to
keep it by the bed."—Age fifty-six.*

*"I was relieved that I couldn't become pregnant again after
four children, and for me sex was better than ever. It was like
a honeymoon for a long time. My husband is a good, considerate lover. He's always wanted a lot of sex. Though since we've
reached our sixties, we seem to be slowing down a little bit. I
never noticed any dryness or changes, and have never had to
use any lubrication."—Age sixty-four.*

*"Lubrication is a problem. I have discomfort and even pain
during intercourse and it's driving me and my husband crazy.
Lubricants help, but are not enough. I'm also prone to yeast
infections. I can't seem to get clear of them. I think my anxiety
about having difficulties feeds on itself, making me more tense*

before intercourse, and causing me more pain. The decline in sexual activity is leaving us both unhappy."—Age forty-nine.

"Yes, I've noticed a little dryness. Sometimes I use a lubricant, and that takes care of it. It hasn't interfered with my sexual enjoyment in the least."—Age sixty-five.

"My vagina feels itchy. And I noticed a decrease in lubrication. But it's not as bad as it used to be. It seems to be getting better. I've heard about using jellies, but I'm not one to try new things. It sounds too gooky."—Age fifty-two.

"My vagina was so painful that it hurt, even when I walked. It was ruining my marriage. Estrogen cream relieved me. And I seem to be lubricating better as I'm getting older."—Age sixty.

There are other changes too: the mons and lips of the vagina lose their fatty padding, so that the clitoris and urethral opening are not as well protected, and may be more vulnerable to irritation. This shouldn't diminish sexual enjoyment—the clitoris is still highly responsive to sexual stimulation. But your partner will have to use more gentle handling during lovemaking.

The ability to have an orgasm, or even multiple orgasms, does not change after menopause. However, with age, the duration and intensity of your orgasms may decrease somewhat. Younger women generally experience five to ten vaginal contractions during sexual climax, while the older woman experiences an average of three to five vaginal contractions.

During an orgasm the uterus of a young woman contracts about three to five times, in a rhythmic fashion. Older women also have uterine contractions, but they are spastic rather than rhythmic. And occasionally, a woman past menopause may feel these contractions as a cramping pain, similar to labor pains.[14,15]

Use It or Lose It

Sex researchers Masters and Johnson studied the sexual responses of sixty-one women between forty and eighty years of age. They discovered that three of these women, all past sixty years of age, lubricated quickly and rapidly, like twenty- to thirty-year-olds, despite the fact that their vaginal walls were very thin. Their orgasms were more intense, and they experienced nearly as many orgasmic contractions as younger women. The secret to their youthful sexual functioning? All three had maintained an active sex life (intercourse at least one to two times a week) throughout their mature adult years. They were the only ones in this study to have maintained sex at that rate.[16]

The conclusion drawn by Masters and Johnson is this: if you don't use it, you'll lose it. Over the years, other research- ers have corroborated this finding. Regular sexual activity, at least once or twice a week, seems to keep the vagina moist and elastic, and more easily lubricated. It also appears to elimi- nate problems with uterine cramping during orgasm. Ac- cording to one medical expert, any kind of sexual arousal which increases blood flow to the area— be it in the form of fantasy, masturbation, intercourse, or even reading or films— will result in improved vaginal health.[17] There is also the pos- sibility that the hormones in a man's ejaculate, when absorbed during intercourse, help to thicken the vaginal walls.

Helping Yourself to a Good Sex Life

The following may help you to maintain a healthy vagina and satisfying sex life.

1. *Gentle, Leisurely Lovemaking.* If you find it takes you longer to lubricate, communicate to your partner the need for more prolonged or imaginative foreplay. When penetra- tion is rushed, intercourse can be uncomfortable, and may even injure sensitive tissues. This may be a golden opportunity to try new, more adventurous approaches in the bedroom.

If you enjoy having your clitoris manipulated during fore- play, or intercourse, you may have to tell your partner to do so more gently. Rough handling can be more irritating than it was before. Vigorous penile thrusting, too, may make you sore. And you may want to experiment with new positions and rhythms that are more comfortable.

2. *Use Additional Lubrication.* Water-soluble lubricants,

such as KY Jelly or contraceptive jellies, can help to alleviate vaginal dryness. Use a lubricant before you have intercourse. Some people incorporate it into their loveplay, applying the jelly to the man's penis, as well as to the woman's vagina. Plain old saliva, which is always on hand and in plentiful supply, is also a good lubricant, as are most vegetable oils. Never use petroleum jelly for this purpose. It can be very irritating to delicate vaginal tissues.

If vaginal dryness is very severe, external lubricants won't provide adequate relief. In such cases, a woman may want to consider taking estrogen, either orally or in vaginal creams or suppositories. Estrogen has been shown to thicken the vaginal lining and increase lubrication. It also creates a more acidic vagina, and it reduces bladder infections and genital irritation. (See Chapter 6 for a complete discussion on the pros and cons of estrogen use.)

Unfortunately, physicians do not yet know of any other alternative treatment for relief of severe vaginal dryness. And women who cannot take estrogen may be placed in a real bind: "I am having a terrible time with vaginal dryness. Intercourse is impossible. I find this highly distressing, and so does my husband. But I just had a mastectomy for breast cancer, and my doctor doesn't want me on estrogen. I don't know what to do."

There are some unorthodox estrogen alternatives mentioned in the lay literature. In her book, *Menopause: A Positive Approach*, Rosetta Reitz suggests yogurt therapy. One tablespoon of yogurt is mixed with one teaspoon of pure, cold-pressed vegetable oil, without preservatives. The mixture is inserted in the vagina once a week, before bedtime, with a plunger applicator used for contraceptive jelly or cream. Reitz recommends that you apply this mixture while lying in bed with a towel spread beneath you. The approach is an admittedly messy one, says the author, but women quickly learn to raise their hips so little of the mixture slides back out.[18]

Maggie Lettvin, an exercise and health enthusiast (*Maggie's Woman's Book*), proposes that a nightly application of Vitamin A and D to the mucous membranes may counteract the thinning, shrinking and drying. She recommends that you squeeze the contents of a cod liver oil capsule in a 5000 A-to-500 D potency onto a piece of cotton and apply it.[19]

Most physicians are skeptical of such therapies. But, concedes one gynecologist, "they may have a healing effect, and they probably won't hurt."

3. *Stay Sexually Active.* Regular sexual activity—at least once or twice a week—helps to keep your vagina more elastic and better lubricated. Whether you achieve orgasm as a result of intercourse or masturbation doesn't make any difference. The main thing is that you contract your pelvic muscles and bring a greater blood flow into the area.

Some people feel inhibited about masturbation, probably because they were cautioned against it as children. There is nothing wrong or harmful about it. Masturbation provides a healthy outlet for sexual tension when you have no partner available, or when your partner isn't "in the mood." And it may help you to discover what pleases you so that you can respond more readily when you do have intercourse. Says one forty-year-old woman: "I was married for sixteen years to a man who made love to me as quickly as possible and then rolled over to sleep. I never had an orgasm and thought there was something wrong with me. After our divorce I began experimenting with masturbation. For the first time in my life I learned how to bring myself to orgasm. Now I know exactly where I like and need to be touched. And, with my new lover, I often have multiple orgasms! I've come alive sexually after all of those wasted years."

Kegel exercises can also improve pelvic muscle tone and sexual enjoyment (see page 187 for more details).

4. *Maintain Good Personal Hygiene.* If you are more prone to vaginal and urinary tract infections now, you may want to take certain preventive measures. Drink plenty of water (at least six to eight glasses) over the course of the day. This will help to cleanse your urinary tract and dilute the bacteria in your urine. Cranberry juice is also recommended because it helps to make urine more acidic.

Always empty your bladder whenever you feel the urge to urinate, and immediately before and after intercourse. Bacterial growth is less likely in an empty bladder. After having a bowel movement, wipe yourself from front to back so that bacteria from your anus doesn't find its way to your vaginal area. During lovemaking, too, take care to wash hands and genitals that have been in contact with anal areas before they touch the vagina or urethra.

Avoid tight underwear or clothing that will rub against your crotch and irritate tender vaginal tissues. Make sure your underwear is made of cotton, which is more soothing to the skin than synthetics. It's also a good idea to sleep without panties, and to choose nightwear that's loose fitting.

Since your vaginal tissues may be especially sensitive, you'll want to avoid cleansing with harsh soaps or soaking in bubble baths. Vaginal sprays and douches can also irritate tender tissues and should not be used unless specifically recommended by your physician.

Sex After Hysterectomy

Some women notice little or no change in their sex lives after having a hysterectomy. A woman can still enjoy sex and experience orgasm without having a uterus or ovaries. When the surgery eliminates profuse bleeding or pain during intercourse, sex will probably be better than it was before. It cannot be denied, however, that 33 to 46 percent of women who undergo this surgery report a decrease in sexual response.[20]

For many years physicians blamed this decrease in sexual interest on psychological factors. Women who felt less sexy after hysterectomy were told that the problem was mainly one of attitude.

There's no doubt that the removal of a woman's womb or ovaries can have powerful effects on her emotions. There are many issues to grapple with after a hysterectomy. Women have to face the fact that they can no longer bear babies. And some feel that the loss of reproductive organs makes them less womanly.

"I'm scheduled for surgery in two weeks—a hysterectomy. I feel as though they're taking away the cradle, the place where I carried my children. My friend who had a hysterectomy says to enjoy it—it will be like a second honeymoon. No more worries about pregnancy. Well, I'd just as soon keep mine."

"*After my surgery, the nurse said to me, 'Why are you so upset? I lost my breast.' But just because the loss is inside of you and you can't see it doesn't mean that you don't feel it as a loss. I grieved for a part of me that was gone. I don't want my periods, but I miss not having the familiar cycles.*"

"*God knew what he was doing when he put it [the uterus] there. It's like a desk that you put together. You may find that you have five screws left over. The desk is still standing, but it's not strong. I'm not the same anymore. I'm different. I'm still standing. But the old person and the new body are at odds. Doctors should be more sensitive to how a woman feels. To me my body is gold—it's not a chicken that you dissect or a frog. It's me. You are taking a part of me, not a diseased tissue. You may be healing my body, but you're ruining my mind.*"

But psychological factors are just one part of the story. The removal of ovaries and/or uterus can upset a woman's delicate hormonal balance and affect her sexuality in subtle ways.

When a woman has her ovaries removed (oophorectomy) estrogen levels plummet and she undergoes what is known as a "surgical" menopause. Hot flashes are likely to be especially severe and vaginal dryness can become a problem. Estrogen therapy corrects these conditions and is usually begun soon after surgery.

But there is one important difference between a surgical menopause and one that occurs naturally: the menopausal woman's ovaries remain intact and continue to produce substantial amounts of male sex hormones. These androgens help to stoke the libido. And their absence after oophorectomy can result in a loss of sexual interest.[21,22,23]

"*I have my ovaries and thought I wasn't supposed to have a decrease in desire. But it happened so suddenly after the operation that I knew it must be connected. I went from a woman who was very sexual to not feeling very desirous at all. This disturbed me. I talked about it to a friend who had the same type of surgery and she confided that she experienced the same feelings. I was so relieved.*"

Androgen therapy has been shown to increase a woman's sexual desire. However, prolonged use of this hormone can permanently virilize a woman, causing such symptoms as a deepening of the voice, excess hair growth and acne. For this reason it is not commonly administered.[24]

The removal of a woman's uterus can also affect her sexual response. According to Masters and Johnson, the uterus is highly responsive throughout all phases of the sex act. Its tissues swell during sexual arousal, and it rises into the pelvic cavity, causing the vagina to balloon out and enlarge. Rhythmic uterine contractions at orgasm contribute to heightened sexual pleasure.[25] When the uterus has been removed, a woman may notice that her orgasms feel less intense, as if less is going on inside of her.

"I've had both my uterus and ovaries removed, and I feel that without uterine contractions my orgasm is not as complete. But there's also something new for me. During orgasm I now can feel a tingling in my legs and toes and body that I never felt before. It's like the rest of me is becoming supersensitive as a compensation for not having a uterus."

Physicians are beginning to suspect that the removal of the uterus causes hormonal changes too. Perhaps this would explain why some hysterectomized women report a diminished sex drive as well as hot flashes and vaginal dryness even though they still have their ovaries. (An alternate explanation is that the blood vessels that nourish the ovaries may be damaged during surgery, causing the ovaries to become dysfunctional.)[26]

According to Dr. Anthony Labrum, a researcher at the University of Rochester School of Medicine, some of the changes caused by a hysterectomy may reverse themselves in time: "When the uterus is removed there is sometimes a temporary decline in blood supply to the ovary. For a brief period of time a woman may experience hot flushes and a sore vagina. But then the blood comes back and the situation reverses itself."

After hysterectomy, some women are afraid that penetration or orgasm might be painful. "If you have a fear of pain," says one sex therapist, "put on a pair of surgical gloves, cover a finger with KY Jelly and insert it into the vagina to see how it feels. If there's enough lubricant, and you are properly healed, it probably won't hurt, and you'll feel more relaxed about having intercourse."

Internal scar tissue can detract from sexual pleasure. When the cervix is removed, the surrounding walls of the vagina must be stitched together. This surgical repair is known as a vaginal cuff. If the cuff has been poorly placed, it may cause pain during intercourse, when the man's penis bumps against the scar tissue. In the rare case of a radical hysterectomy, the vagina may be significantly shortened. And this, too, can make intercourse uncomfortable.

External scars can also generate concerns: "After surgery I was left with a big, ugly scar from my navel to my pubic hair. I worried, would it turn my husband off?" "Nobody's perfect," observes the sex therapist. "Not your body, nor the man's. Stand together in front of a mirror in the nude and look at each other, and you'll see that this is the case. I had one of my patients, who had a mastectomy, do this exercise with her husband. It helped them to diffuse the issue, and got them to look at themselves on a deeper level—the love of a person versus the love of their body parts. This can lead to a deepening relationship."

The way a woman will react to sex after hysterectomy depends on a combination of physical and psychological factors. The woman who has a good self-image and a positive attitude about sex, is, no doubt, one step ahead of the game. If she has very active adrenal glands, pumping plenty of androgens into her bloodstream, then she may notice no lack in sexual interest despite the fact that she's had an oophorectomy. Some women are apparently less attuned than others to uterine changes during sexual arousal and orgasm; for them, the lack of a uterus is less likely to detract from the quality of sex.

A supportive, nonpressuring mate, who is willing to take the time to arouse and stimulate his partner, makes post-surgery adjustments easier, and allows a woman to more fully enjoy whatever sexual capacity she has.

Sex and the Single Woman

Though most women are willing and able to have sexual relations into their middle years, circumstances may deny them ample opportunity. Divorce is common in the middle years and widowhood is the rule rather than the exception: three out of every four women will ultimately outlive their mates.[27] The ratio of eligible males to females decreases as a woman ages, and the likelihood of remarriage also declines.

A woman can be thrust quite suddenly from a secure, familiar marital relationship to a world of single dances and dates. One social worker who leads a support group for older singles makes these observations:

"Many of the women in my group think it's wrong to enjoy sex in their fifties. So they desensitize themselves and deny their sexuality. They are afraid of being exploited in a sexual relationship. Yet if they enjoy sex and a man's companionship, too, they are, in a sense 'using' men. It's like going through a second adolescence, but there are life experiences in between that cannot be denied."

Several women describe how they feel about dating and sexuality after widowhood or divorce:

"I don't think that my desire or need for sexuality has decreased. But it's very hard to find a man. I have a lot of friends and we go out together in groups. We've tried all of the dances and singles groups. It's good to get out. But it sometimes feels so awkward. If no one asks you to dance it's hard not to feel rejected."—Age fifty-five.

"My husband passed away seven years ago. He was a unique man. And I was madly in love with him. I don't sit around depressed. I keep very busy and am working, and doing a lot of volunteer work. I occasionally like to go out with a man for dinner and to have good company. But I'm not interested in getting sexually involved or marrying again. Friends say I'm comparing too much. Yes, I do compare. I can't help it."— Age sixty-three.

"I've always enjoyed sex, and the lack of a regular sex life

since my divorce is very upsetting to me. I've gone to just about every singles bar, and there are always five attractive single women to every man. The competition is fierce. And the middle-aged guys are going for the younger women. I've even taken to answering personal ads in a local singles publication. Typically the ads read something like this: '50-year-old man seeks attractive 30-year-old female—preferably without dependent children.' They want to have their cake and eat it too. And it seems as if they're getting it."—Age forty-four.

"My husband died over thirty years ago. I've never remarried. I never did have a high sex drive. I had one slight affair with one man and I found I was not sexually aroused. My sexual desire is petering out. There's dryness and it's painful. The doctor said to use KY Jelly to relieve the dryness. But there's no reason to get into that. I don't want to be involved with anyone sexually. I like to go out socially, to have a nice dinner, but not to go to bed with anyone."—Age sixty-five.

"I've had no lack of dates since my divorce. Men seem to be crawling out of the woodwork. They all want me to go to bed with them and to be instantly orgasmic. When they find out that I have two young kids they run with their tails between their legs. It's like being a teenager all over again. Does he really like me? Will he call? I feel confused and vulnerable. And easily hurt. I'm too old to be playing these emotional games."—Age thirty-eight.

If sex is only a once-in-a-while thing, it can be uncomfortable, especially if a woman hasn't been masturbating regularly. The vagina shrinks with disuse and doesn't lubricate as quickly or completely. This is true no matter what a woman's age, though the older the woman, the more pronounced the changes, and the harder it will probably be to reverse them.[28] A lover has to be gentle and patient until the vagina gradually becomes more flexible. External lubricants may be helpful. However, if the woman is past menopause, and finds sex to be extremely painful, she may find it necessary to use estrogen.

Contraception

So long as you are having periods—no matter how erratic or far apart they occur—you can still become pregnant. If you don't want to conceive, you should use some form of birth control for at least one full year after your periods stop. If you are still in your forties, some doctors even suggest that you use some form of contraception for two years, just to play it safe.

Generally speaking, the "pill" is not recommended for women over thirty-five, because it is associated with an increased risk of heart disease and stroke among this age group.

If you've been using an IUD, you may be able to leave it in place until you're sure you are no longer fertile. However, an IUD must be removed if irregular or prolonged and heavy bleeding occurs. These symptoms can be a normal reaction to the hormonal changes of menopause, but they can also be signs of more serious problems.

Couples who have used natural family planning in the past may find it increasingly difficult to do so around menopause. Periods may become irregular, and the texture of the cervical mucous may change, making it more difficult to figure out when ovulation is occurring. If pregnancy is not desired, the couple may have to consider using another form of birth control.

Barrier methods, such as diaphragm, condom and contraceptive foams, are effective and safe, and women who are comfortable with these methods may continue using them.

Sterilization has become the contraceptive method of choice in this country. Tubal ligation for women, and vasectomy for men, can both be done in a doctor's office, or on an outpatient basis. Both are highly effective, and so far seem to entail little risk. You may want to consider this if you are in your thirties or early forties. But there *are* some drawbacks. Both procedures, at the current time, are largely irreversible. So if the sterilized person decides to have children at a later date it will not be possible. Some women experience heavy and irregular menstrual bleeding and cramping following tubal ligation. And some studies show a link between female sterilization and higher rates of hysterectomies and premature menopause. These changes may be brought about by injuries to the blood vessels leading to the ovaries. Men who have had vasectomies appear to develop a high number of antibodies to their own sperm. What this means in terms of future health—if anything—is not yet known.[29,30]

Often women who become pregnant in their later years opt for an abortion. When performed in the early months, abortion is a safe and relatively simple medical procedure.

Today it is not unusual for a woman to postpone childbearing until her late thirties or early forties. It is certainly possible to have a normal, healthy pregnancy at this time, although the chances of birth defects and pregnancy complications do increase with age. It becomes especially important to receive good prenatal care. Most doctors recommend that pregnant women thirty-five and over have an amniocentesis. Amniotic fluid is removed through a hollow needle and studied in the lab to identify certain potential birth defects.

Male Sexual Response

Nature seems to have played a nasty prank on men and women. In his teens, a man is in his sexual heyday. His hormones course through his veins with a Niagara-like rush. As one man laughingly recalls: "I spent half my high school life with an erection, afraid the teacher would call on me and that I'd have to stand up for all my classmates to see." By eighteen years of age, a man is considered to be at his sexual zenith. After that his libido gradually tapers off.

Enter the sexually inexperienced young woman. She is more likely to start her sexual life off in the slow lane. Perhaps it's a result of cultural expectations and the double standard, but a teenage female is not usually as sexually driven as her masculine counterpart. She may feel that young men are too pushy and eager, and don't take enough time. With increased experience the young woman becomes more easily aroused and primed for orgasm. Most women reach their sexual peak in their late thirties and forties—the time at which a man's sexual capabilities begin to wane. Biologically speaking, a forty-year-old woman is most sexually compatible with young men half her age.

"There is less sexual interest on his part, while mine is very strong. When my husband is responsive, sex is highly pleasurable for me. His lack of desire is a great source of anxiety and frustration to me. I have a fear that I'm less attractive to my husband than I used to be."—A woman in her late forties.

The disharmony between men and women usually eases up when a couple enters their fifties or sixties. While sex still remains an important part of their lives, men and women may find that their sex drives become less urgent.[31]

"I have always had a higher sex drive than my husband. We are not matched as well as we might be. As my libido decreases it's helpful. Our relationship is better in so many ways. My husband is a tender and good lover."—Age fifty-five.

Changes in sexual anatomy and functioning are natural and occur in everyone with advancing age. The physical similarities between men and women are actually very striking.

Men, like women, lose elasticity in their genitalia. Scrotal tissue may sag and fold with advancing age, and the testicular swelling that occurs in a young man during sex is less likely to occur once a man passes his mid-fifties.

Lubrication is the first sign of sexual arousal in a woman. An erection is its male equivalent. Both take longer to occur with age. A young man can become hard in seconds, at just the fleeting thought of sex. But a man in his fifties or sixties may take minutes to become erect. And he may need more direct stimulation from his partner than before. The erection may not be as high and firm as it used to be, especially if the man is over sixty years of age.

But age has its rewards too. Once an older man becomes erect, he can stay that way for a long period of time without ejaculating. This increased staying power presents opportunities for lengthy sessions of foreplay. And an older lover has plenty of time to bring his partner to orgasm before he satisfies himself.

The young man has a two stage orgasm: he first senses that ejaculation is about to occur (for two to three seconds), and then he loses control and ejaculates. The older man may lose the first stage and find that he ejaculates with little or no prior warning at all. Or else he may find that the warning stage lasts twice as long as usual.

The volume of seminal fluid decreases, and it is expelled with less force. Occasionally, the semen may just seep out, or the sex act may end with no ejaculation at all. According to Masters and Johnson, the average sixty-year-old has sex once or twice a week and may ejaculate every second or third time. The number of orgasmic contractions also declines; and by the time a man is over sixty, he may have only one or two contractions during orgasm.[32]

Repeat performances are usual for a young man, who may remain swollen for minutes, or even hours after orgasm, and have several erections during the course of one lovemaking session. This is not so for the older man. The ability to regain an erection lengthens with age, and instead of minutes, it may take hours—and sometimes an entire day—before he can have another. If he is over sixty, sexual resolution may occur so quickly that his penis returns to a flaccid state within seconds, sometimes falling right out of the vagina. This can be quite alarming for both partners if they don't realize that it is a very natural occurrence.

Of course, these changes vary from man to man, and even from one sexual encounter to another. Some men will notice a change in sexual functioning in their forties or fifties while others retain their youthful functioning far longer. In men, as in women, there is a "use it or lose it" phenomenon. Men who have frequent sex throughout their adult lives are less likely to have problems achieving and maintaining an erection in their later years.

Adapting to Sexual Changes

Changes in male sexuality are very gradual and are not marked by a concrete event like menopause. There is some controversy over whether these changes are caused by a decline in the male hormone testosterone or by the natural process of aging.[33,34] Very little research has been done on hormone therapy for men.

In many ways, a man has more sexual adjustments to contend with after fifty than a woman does. Females are always in a state of sexual readiness and may have sex repeatedly. But a man may have obvious difficulty achieving an erection, or regaining it once it is lost. He may see this as a sign of declining virility, and may worry himself into a state of impotence. By trying too hard to force an erection, a man may find he has ever-increasing trouble attaining one. Some begin to avoid sex altogether, or else try to prove themselves by having extramarital affairs.

A man's increased response time or failure to ejaculate is sometimes misinterpreted by his partner. She may think that her husband no longer finds her attractive or that she is not a good enough lover. The plain truth is, he needs more direct stimulation than when he was younger. A wife may try to tiptoe around her husband's ego by remaining silent and making as few sexual demands as possible, but it would be better all around if both discussed their feelings in the open. Communication between two partners is very important during these times of changing sexuality.

Sometimes a couple has to move away from their traditional definitions of sex. A man and woman do not always have to achieve orgasm to have good sex. And sex can be joyous even when penetration isn't possible. Touching, caressing, licking and nibbling can create wonderfully erotic sensations. And close physical contact presents an opportunity for renewed intimacy.

Special Problems

Most men experience impotence at some time in their lives. Mental and physical fatigue can cause it. And so can emotional upsets. If a man is overly preoccupied by problems at the work place or with family crises, his sex life is likely to be temporarily upset.

Overindulgence in food and alcohol can cause impotence at any age. And certain drugs, such as blood pressure medication, barbiturates and tranquilizers, can adversely affect sexual desire and performance in both men and women.[35] (If you suspect a prescription drug is affecting you or your spouse sexually, discuss it with your physician. Often the dosage can be lowered or the drug changed to alleviate the problem.)

Sometimes the problem is simply one of boredom. Sexual routines may need shaking up after many years of marriage. And you both may want to experiment with lotions, vibrators and new techniques and positions. (For some ideas you can consult a sex guide, such as *For Yourself: The Fulfillment of Female Sexuality* by Lonnie Garfield Barbach.) If there are children living at home, try to arrange an occasional getaway weekend where just the two of you can focus on each other.

The incidence of illness does increase in the middle years. Yet all but the most severe usually allow for continued physical intimacy on some level. Don't hesitate to discuss frankly with your physician how a particular medical problem may affect your sex life.

A normal, active sex life is usually possible after a heart attack, and may even facilitate recovery.[36] Sex is also possible in cases of arthritis and stroke, though a couple may have to experiment with different positions and, in the case of arthritis, have sex during times when pain is least likely to flare up.

Diabetes is one of the few diseases that may cause permanent sexual impairment. When it strikes after age fifty it can cause impotence in a man and a lack of lubrication and clitoral response in a woman. Counseling and therapy may not be as effective in correcting the situation as it is among younger people stricken with this disease.[37]

Physical changes caused by surgery may influence the way a man or woman feels about sex. After prostate surgery, it is common for the semen to ejaculate inwardly, and a man may think he's impotent, though this isn't really the case.[38]

A woman who has had a mastectomy may have fears about her sexual attractiveness. And both she and her partner may benefit from mastectomy support groups and counseling services offered through the American Cancer Society. Says one woman of her mastectomy: "After the operation I almost died when I first took off the bandage. I looked so ugly. But Lou has always been very good about it, and still seems to find me attractive. He keeps saying that it's me that he loves and not just my body. I'm the one who has trouble accepting it. Not one day passes where I don't remember I have a deformity. I put my prosthesis on the minute I wake up, and I wear it when we're making love."

When poor sex becomes a continuing problem, no matter what the reason, a man or woman should seek outside help. It's important to first be examined by a physician to rule out any physical problems. However, according to one sex counselor, your doctor is not likely to be the best authority on human sexuality. "Doctors may not be knowledgeable in this area. They may tell the patient nothing's wrong, or nothing can be done." In fact, some doctors do not feel comfortable about discussing sex with their patients.

"In my experience after surgery, the doctor paced back and forth smoking cigarettes, visibly tense. As he went out the door he poked his head in and said, 'By the way, no more relations until six weeks.' 'What about friends?' my husband joked. That seemed to break the ice. The doctor laughed and came back into the room and sat down and was able to talk to us about it."

The best source of advice on sexual problems is a sex therapist or counselor. You might try contacting one through a family services agency, Planned Parenthood or your local mental health center. Some religious agencies also provide this type of counseling. You may also want to write to the American Association of Sex Educators, Counselors and Therapists (see the back of this book for the address). They publish a National Register of Certified Sex Educators and Sex Therapists.

Every healthy man and woman has the capacity for sex well into ripe old age. And everyone is entitled to enjoy to the fullest this aspect of their lives. Even when faced with physical problems, there is often a way to receive and give some form of sexual pleasure.

Chapter 10
Body
Changes

"My hair is a nice shade of gray. People compliment me on it. I haven't minded the gray hairs at all. But the wrinkles are hard. I understand why aging actresses go in for plastic surgery. They have to look in the mirror all the time. I feel like I'm a young woman inside. The wrinkles are kind of a shock."—Age fifty-five.

"Our culture puts such stress on youth. You feel that maybe this bulge or wrinkle shouldn't be there. My daughter doesn't like me looking older. She wants me to be more glamorous. She told me I should color my hair. At first I did. But then I said, to heck with this. I'm a more natural type. This is the way I am."—Age fifty-six.

"I feel angry when I see ads for Oil of Olay. As if that one little drop is going to do it all."—Age forty-seven.

Aging begins at birth. And certain normal changes are bound to become noticeable as you reach your middle years. Internal organs, skin, hair, teeth and eyes—all are affected by the passage of time. Menopause may have some influence on these changes. But it can't be blamed for all of the natural consequences of aging.

Pelvic Organs

Approximately half of all women are affected to some degree by a condition known as pelvic relaxation.[1] The muscles and tissues in the pelvic area become stretched out and weak. They may not be able to adequately support the bladder, urethra, rectum and uterus. And these organs may begin to sag.

One of the first signs of weak pelvic muscles may be the involuntary escape of urine whenever a woman laughs, coughs, sneezes or does any strenuous lifting or exercise. In medical terms, this inability to hold urine is known as stress incontinence. When it becomes a constant occurrence, it can be a terrible source of social embarrassment. Some women find it necessary to wear sanitary pads every day in order to protect their clothing.

Another sign of weak pelvic muscles may be the loss of sensation during intercourse. The penis may feel as if it is lost inside of the vagina.

Some women seem to be born with a tendency toward weak pelvic muscles. But pelvic relaxation is more likely the result of injuries during the normal course of childbirth. Though the actual damage occurs at the time of birth, symptoms do not usually show up until after menopause. Prolonged periods of standing, chronic coughing, heavy lifting and constant straining at the toilet all aggravate this condition. So may obesity. Menopause and aging together help to worsen the situation because they make supporting tissues thinner and less elastic.

In extreme cases the pelvic tissues and muscles become so stretched out that the fibers separate, and a hole is eventually created. The pelvic organs may protrude, or prolapse, through the defect and bulge into the vaginal wall. These prolapsed organs are, in effect, vaginal hernias. The following is a brief rundown of various prolapse conditions:

- *Urethrocele:* The urethra is the tube that connects the bladder to the urinary opening. When it protrudes into the vaginal wall the condition is known as a urethrocele. Poor bladder control may result from this condition.
- *Cystocele:* A cystocele occurs when the urinary bladder sags into the vaginal canal. If the prolapse is mild, there may be no symptoms. A more extreme prolapse may make it difficult for a woman to completely empty her bladder each time she urinates. This means that a residual amount of urine is left in the bladder and may be the source of frequent infections. A woman with a cystocele may experience a heavy, dragging sensation in her pelvic area. Her bladder capacity is reduced, so she constantly feels as if she has to go to the bathroom—even after she has just urinated. In severe cases a bulge or lump can be felt inside the vagina. Some find that by pushing up on this bulge with their fingers, they can more completely empty their bladders.
- *Rectocele:* This condition develops when the rectum sags into the back wall of the vagina. Stools tend to get trapped and harden in the rectal outpouchings. And chronic constipation may become a problem. A finger in the vagina against the rectal wall may assist in more fully emptying the bowels. And care should be taken in the diet to help keep stools soft.
- *Prolapsed Uterus:* Also known as a "dropped" uterus. The muscles and ligaments that hold the uterus in place weaken, usually due to childbirth, and the uterus sags into the vaginal canal. There are varying degrees of severity. In first-degree uterine prolapse, the uterus is sagging but does not yet protrude through the vaginal opening, and there may be few symptoms. Second-degree prolapse means that part of the uterus may appear outside of the vagina. Third-degree prolapse is when the entire uterus comes through the vaginal opening.

The prolapsed uterus can pull the bladder, urethra or rectum down along with it, causing urinary and bowel problems. And a woman may experience backaches and a sensation of heaviness in her pelvic area. When standing, some say they

The Uterus, Fallopian Tubes and Ovaries

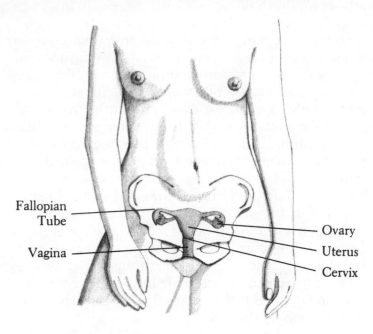

Fallopian Tube

Vagina

Ovary

Uterus

Cervix

External female anatomy

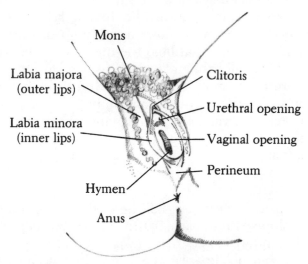

Mons

Labia majora (outer lips)

Labia minora (inner lips)

Clitoris

Urethral opening

Vaginal opening

Perineum

Hymen

Anus

feel as if their internal organs are dropping out. Often a woman's sex partner is the first one to notice that her uterus is prolapsed. He can feel it during intercourse. In rare cases a woman may actually see her uterus protruding from her vagina.

Estrogen therapy cannot cure pelvic relaxation. But it may help to alleviate symptoms by thickening the vaginal and urinary tract linings. When a woman's symptoms are so severe that they interfere with her normal daily activities, surgery may be recommended to repair weakened walls and reposition the bladder, urethra or rectum. If the uterus has descended completely into the vagina, a hysterectomy may be the only recourse. The hysterectomy is usually performed through the vagina, and repairs to the bladder or rectum may be done at the same time, if need be.

Sometimes severe health problems make a hysterectomy undesirable. In such cases a doctor may fit a woman with a rubber or plastic device called a pessary. The device fits around the cervix and holds the uterus and other organs in place. It is not a good permanent solution, however, as it is hard to properly fit, and tends to cause irritations and unpleasant-smelling vaginal discharge. The pessary is also a potential source of infection and has to be removed, cleaned and reinserted by a physician every few months.

Fortunately, pelvic relaxation is usually mild and simple exercises designed to strengthen pelvic muscles may be all that are needed to improve the condition. Surgery is necessary in fewer than 10 percent of all cases.[2]

Kegel Exercises

Kegel exercises, named after the physician who invented them, are aimed at strengthening your pubococcygeal muscles. This band of muscles stretches tightly between your legs, from your pubic bone to your coccyx. Like a sling, it holds your organs firmly in place, and fits snugly around your urethra, anus and vagina. (See illustration on page 189.) You can easily locate these muscles by voluntarily stopping and starting a flow of urine at midstream.

NORMAL VIEW

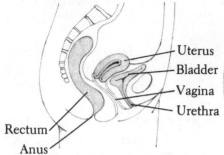

Uterus
Bladder
Vagina
Urethra
Rectum
Anus

Cystocele
(prolapse of the bladder)

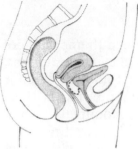

Rectocele
(prolapse of the rectum)

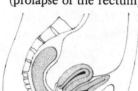

Urethrocele
(prolapse of the urethra)

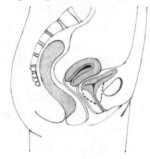

Uterine Prolapse
("dropped" uterus)

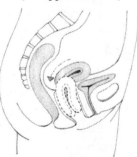

Vaginal Pessary

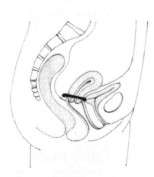

The Pubococcygeal Muscle

By exercising the pubococcygeal muscle daily, you can improve bladder control and help prevent organs from sagging into the vagina.

SIDE VIEW

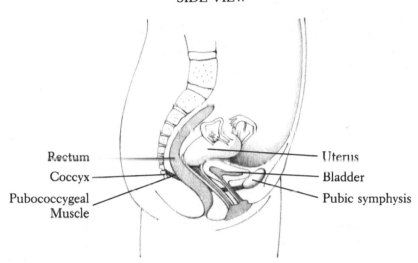

Rectum

Coccyx

Pubococcygeal
Muscle

Uterus

Bladder

Pubic symphysis

TOP VIEW

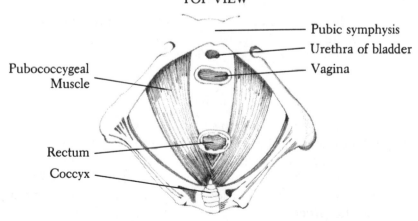

Pubococcygeal
Muscle

Rectum

Coccyx

Pubic symphysis

Urethra of bladder

Vagina

Kegel exercises are done by alternately tightening and relaxing the pubococcygeal muscles. When you tighten the muscle, hold it for three seconds, and then relax it for the same amount of time. You should feel as if you are drawing your anus and genitals upward together. (Do not bear down as for a bowel movement. There should be no straining, and you should be breathing naturally.) You can tell if you are doing Kegels correctly if you feel your vagina tighten around an inserted finger.

The more contractions you do a day, the better. As with any exercise, you may want to build up your muscles gradually. Perhaps you can start by doing twenty a day at first, and slowly work your way up to one hundred. You can do them in groups of ten throughout the day, or all at once.

Kegels can be done in any position, anywhere, anytime and no one will be any the wiser. You may practice them while riding home from work on the bus, for example, or while standing on line at the bank. To be effective, however, they must be done conscientiously every day.

In many cases, Kegels can improve or eliminate problems with stress incontinence. They help strengthen support of the bladder, urethra and rectum, and may forestall the need for surgery in later years. By tightening vaginal muscles, Kegels may also increase sexual sensation and pleasure. These changes will not occur overnight, though. It may take two to three months of regular exercise before you see tangible results.

If you find that you are having problems with bladder control you should not neglect to consult your physician. Infections or other problems may cause similar symptoms, and may need immediate treatment.

Skin

We can often judge a person's age by his skin. We don't really expect a middle-aged woman's skin to look like a young girl's. Yet, each year, Americans spend millions on cosmetics that promise to turn back the biologic time clock. The truth of the matter is, no skin cream or lotion has yet been made that can reverse the process of aging.

Your skin is the largest organ in your body, and it is the only organ that is completely exposed to the external environment. It is made up of several layers. The epidermis is the uppermost skin layer. It constantly replaces itself, as cells from below divide, move to the surface and flake off. The dermis, or second layer, contains collagen and elastic fibers. These give the skin its shape and springy resilience. An underlying third layer consists of fatty tissue which helps the skin to look smooth.

As the skin ages, certain predictable changes take place. The production of new skin cells slows down, and the epidermis can't replace itself as quickly. The supporting fibers in the dermis break down and lose elasticity—which means that skin begins to wrinkle and sag. And there is a decrease in the number of oil and sweat glands, so that skin is not as moist or well-lubricated. The fatty layer below the dermis also diminishes, changing the contour of the face. Older skin is usually thinner and dryer. It may be more easily damaged or irritated and slower to heal. Sometimes the dryness causes an annoying itchiness.

Does menopause make the skin age faster? This is extremely difficult for scientists to verify.[3] Declining estrogen levels at menopause do seem to accelerate the skin's aging process somewhat. Estrogen therapy may give the skin a slightly fuller look. But to blame aging skin entirely on menopause is unrealistic. It is just one of many contributing factors—including cigarette smoking, alcohol consumption, heredity, exposure to the environment, nutrition and lifestyle.

Wrinkle Prevention

Why is it that some people wrinkle sooner than others? To some extent, it's just the luck of the genetic draw. Cigarette smoking cuts oxygen circulation to the skin, and ups your odds of wrinkling. And rapid weight loss adds more to the ante. The single most important contribution to wrinkled skin, however, is too much sun.

That healthy looking tan you worked on all summer may not really be so healthy at all. It's true that your body needs a certain amount of sun in order to manufacture vitamin D.

But excessive exposure to ultraviolet rays causes skin to sag and wrinkle before its time. And worse, it's the leading cause of skin cancer. An estimated 300,000 cases of this disease each year are the result of too much sun.

The sun attacks the skin on two fronts. It thickens the dermis, or upper layer, and it damages the elastic fibers that support it from underneath. This damage doesn't show up at first. It is slow and cumulative. Over many years of constant exposure the skin becomes tough, leathery, yellow and dry. Wrinkles and lines form on the face, neck and hands.

The sun is also responsible for deepening pigmented areas and creating "old age freckles" or "liver spots." Squinting from bright sunlight contributes to crow's feet.

Fair-skinned, blue-eyed people are most susceptible to sun damage, especially if they live in hot, sunny climates or work outdoors. Those with darker complexions are better protected by extra melanin, or skin pigment. Their skin doesn't burn as easily and generally remains younger looking longer. However, people of all skin types, both fair and dark, should take care to avoid excessive sunbathing.

Perhaps Southern belles of the past had the right idea to use sun parasols to keep their complexions creamy. You, too, should make an effort to guard your skin against sun damage. Try to avoid sunbathing when the sun's rays are the strongest—between 10 A.M. and 2 P.M. If you have to be out in the sun, protect your face and neck with a brimmed hat or visor. And use dark glasses to prevent squinting. The best protection of all is a sunscreen, applied liberally to all areas of your body not covered by clothing. (If you're going to wear makeup, apply sunscreen under it first.) Easily burned types may also want to use zinc oxide cream on sensitive areas like the nose and lips.

Sunscreens contain an ingredient—usually PABA (para-aminobenzic acid)—that scatter or absorb the ultraviolet light rays. They are labeled by their manufacturers with Sun Protection Factor (SPF) numbers, ranging from 2 to 15. The higher the number, the more protection a particular sunscreen offers. To be most effective, sunscreens should be applied at least one half hour before you go out in the sun, and reapplied after swimming or perspiring.

Be aware that certain drugs can combine with the sun to make skin more sensitive than usual to ultraviolet light. These include tranquilizers, antiemetics (to prevent vomiting), diuretics, blood pressure medications, sulfa drugs, oral diabetic drugs, tetracycline antibiotics and quinidine (a medication used to stop irregularities of the heartbeat).[4]

Sunlamps and tanning salons that give a fashionable year-round tan also give a liberal dose of damaging ultraviolet rays and are best avoided.

Breasts

The skin on your breasts is no different from the skin on the rest of your body. It too becomes thinner, dryer and less resilient as you age. The muscles and ligaments that support the breasts also become less elastic, and the breasts begin to droop. A good supportive bra may help prevent the stretching of breast ligaments. But much depends on heredity and the shape of your breasts. Small-breasted women are less likely to sag than large-breasted women. And broad-based breasts will keep their shape longer than narrow-based breasts.

Changes also occur inside the breast. Each breast is made up of milk-producing glands surrounded by protective fatty tissue. It is the fat that gives the breast its size and determines its shape. The glands themselves take up relatively little space. During the reproductive years, these glands are extremely responsive to estrogen. They swell just before you menstruate, and during pregnancy and lactation. After menopause, when the breasts no longer have to prepare for pregnancy, the milk glands shrink. Fat tissue is replaced by fibrous tissue. So the breasts become smaller, flatter and softer than before.

Though breasts generally decrease in size as women age, some swear that they've had just the opposite experience: "I used to wear falsies," says one sixty-two-year-old. "Now I look better than ever." Says a sixty-five-year-old: "When I was younger I didn't wear a bra. Now my breasts seem bigger to me, and they're drooping." Breasts may appear bigger because they have become more pendulous. Or the increase in breast size may reflect a gain in weight.

Dry Skin

At around the age of forty, many women begin to notice that their skin is a bit dryer than usual. This tendency toward dry skin usually increases after menopause, when oil and sweat glands function less efficiently. While dryness isn't the cause of wrinkles, it can accentuate them and make your skin look older. Now is the time to pamper your skin, paying attention to its needs for extra moisture.

The following are some common-sense tips on dry skin care:

• Protect your skin from extreme cold and windy weather by covering up with clothing. Use moisturizers on exposed body parts and petroleum jelly on lips to prevent them from cracking.

• Don't bathe to excess. Daily bathing robs the skin of its protective surface oils. Instead, take sponge baths a few times a week. And when you do bathe, make baths and showers brief. Keep your bath water on the lukewarm side. Water that is too hot opens your pores and increases moisture loss.

Bath oils are good for dry skin. You can soak in them, or apply them to a wet washcloth at the end of a bath or shower before you pat yourself dry.

• Use soaps sparingly. They are very drying to skin. Deodorant soaps are probably the most irritating of all. A better choice would be a soap containing cold cream (like Dove or Camay) or a superfatted soap with little or no fragrance. If you have very sensitive skin you may want to use a soap substitute (such as Lowila or Emulave). These won't lather as well, but they are nonirritating. One beauty adviser who runs her own cosmetics company tells her clients to stay away from soaps completely. She recommends instead a milky cleansing lotion.

• Dry skin is generally worse in winter weather. Not only do the cold temperature and wind outdoors dry your skin, but indoor heating, combined with low humidity, decrease your skin's ability to retain moisture. A humidifier will help to alleviate these drying conditions. You may want to use one nightly over the winter months. (Humidifiers, if not properly washed out each week, can be a breeding place for unhealthy funguses and molds. So make sure you follow manufacturer's directions and clean it regularly.)

• Wear cotton-lined rubber gloves to protect your hands when you wash dishes or use any household detergents or chemicals. You might want to keep a jar of hand lotion near the sink, and apply it when you finish working in the kitchen.

• Fingernails, like skin, have a tendency to become dry and brittle as you age. They also grow more slowly than before. Hand lotions and soaking in olive oil will help to keep them more resilient. If you like to keep your nails lacquered, try not to change nail polish too frequently. Both the polish and remover have a drying effect. Touch up any small chips in lieu of repolishing. This will prove far less damaging to your nails.

• Healthy skin reflects good nutrition. Eat a well-balanced diet and drink plenty of liquids. Pay special attention to foods rich in vitamins, A, B, D and E. (Refer to the vitamin chart in Chapter 7.)

• Use moisturizing creams and lotions daily.

Moisturizers and Wrinkle Creams

Hundreds of products promise to banish wrinkles and keep you looking eternally young. In actuality, no cream has yet been developed that can penetrate your skin and undo the damages of time.

All moisturizers are a blend of three basic ingredients: oil, wax and water. They work by forming an oily film over the skin, preventing your body's moisture from evaporating into the air. When a moisturizer contains more water than oil, it is usually called a lotion. If there is more oil in it than water, it is commonly referred to as a cream. The higher the oil content, the thicker the moisturizer is, and the better it coats the skin and retards moisture loss.

The best moisturizers are not necessarily the most expensive. In fact one of the least expensive—petroleum jelly—works just fine. For aesthetic reasons, many women prefer to apply the more effective, but greasier preparations at bedtime, and the lighter, more pleasing textured lotions in the morning.

Moisturizers work best when they are applied over damp

skin. So wet your skin with a compress first, dab it dry, and then smooth on the lotion or cream. One of the best times to apply face and body moisturizers is just after you've had a bath or shower, while your skin is still damp.

What about those expensive wrinkle creams that contain estrogen, collagen or other exotic ingredients? According to the experts, the only benefits from such rejuvenating creams are the temporary relief from dryness that they provide. If they do minimize wrinkles, it's only because of the moisturizers they contain. [5,6,7]

Nor is there any proof that facial exercises, masks or scrubs will help to prevent or reverse aging. They may make your skin feel tingly and look tighter, but the results are only temporary. [8] "That may be true," concedes one cosmetologist, "but facials do give you a psychological lift. Your skin feels as if it's glowing, and it looks great even if only for a few hours. It's a nice way to refresh your face before going out for the evening."

If you want a temporary morale boost, then beauty facials may give them to you. The only permanent way to eliminate wrinkles and sagging skin, however, is through cosmetic surgery.

Cosmetic Surgery

Once confined to the rich and famous, cosmetic surgery is filtering down to the rest of the population. More and more "everyday" people are undergoing operations in the hopes of looking more youthful. Plastic surgery can be expensive and if done for purely cosmetic reasons will not be covered under most medical plans. The most common types of facial surgery to banish wrinkles and aging skin are as follows:

Face Lifts

An incision is made along the hairline and in front of and behind the ears. The skin is then stretched, trimmed where necessary, repositioned and sewn back in place. The procedure requires several days' hospitalization. Swelling and discoloration usually subside within two weeks. Scars, camou-

Cosmetic Surgery

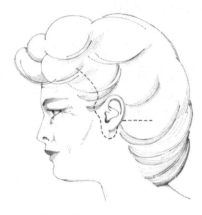

Face lift

Eyelid tuck

flaged by hair and facial folds, should become less noticeable over time.

Face lifts help to eliminate saggy folds, and make the skin look more elastic. But they don't help as much with wrinkles around the eyes, mouth, forehead and brows. After a successful face lift a person may look five or even ten years younger than before. How long the effects will last depend upon a person's individual aging pattern, as well as on the amount of exposure to sun, alcohol and cigarettes (all of which tend to age the skin). Ideally, a face lift should last from five to ten years. Repeated face lifts may give the skin an unnatural texture.

People who have had this operation are advised to keep a constant weight level. Their skin is less elastic, and should they gain and then lose a great deal of weight, it will stretch, fold and sag. One possible complication of the operation is injury to facial nerves, which can leave an area of the face

weak and droopy. (Sometimes this weakness is only temporary.) While people continue to age at their normal pace after
a face lift, they always look younger than they would have
without surgery.

Eyelid Tucks

As a person's face ages, the upper eyelids tend to lose elasticity and droop, and accumulated fat causes bags to form
around the eyes. Eyelid tucks eliminate these problems. An
incision is made along the crease of the upper lid and just
below the lashes of the lower lid. Then extra skin and fat are
removed and the skin is sewn back in place. Since the skin is
stretched less than it is in a face lift, the results of this operation are longer lasting. Eyelid tucks require a one-day hospital stay. Swelling and discoloration caused by the procedure
usually subside within ten to fourteen days.

Skin Peeling

This technique is used on wrinkled skin around the mouth,
forehead and eyes. It is actually a controlled second-degree
chemical burn. Caustic agents are used to destroy areas of
the epidermis and uppermost dermis so that new skin can
form. A person will develop wrinkles in the new skin over time.
How quickly depends upon the individual's rate of aging.
There are some possible complications: The area which has
been peeled may take on a darker or lighter pigmentation than
the rest of the face and, if the burn goes too deep, permanent
scarring can result. People who undergo a skin peel must stay
out of the sun to avoid discoloration of the new skin.

Dermabrasion

This is the mechanical counterpart of the skin peel. Wrinkled areas are removed by abrasion with a rapidly rotating wire
brush. Skin swelling may be severe for a day or two, and resulting scabs usually take ten to fourteen days to heal. Though
the process is a little safer than chemical peeling, the results
may not be as even. There is also the possibility of scarring.
And, as in face peeling, new skin must be protected from
pigmentation by the sun.

There are those who have unrealistic expectations about

what plastic surgery can do for them. They may expect it to solve their marital problems, for example, or to help them get ahead at the work place. While cosmetic surgery may make a woman appear younger, she still has to come to grips with the fact that she is aging. Looking younger is entirely different from being younger.

Some women feel better about themselves after cosmetic surgery. They consider the psychological boost to be well worth the discomfort and expense. Others see facial lines as proof of their experience and maturity, and opt to grow old graciously.

The choice to have—or not to have—plastic surgery is a very individual matter. As with all surgery, there are always possible risks and complications; these should be thoroughly discussed ahead of time with your surgeon.

Growths and Age Spots

As you enter your forties and fifties you may begin to notice new skin blemishes and growths that you never had before. These are due to changes in hormones, oil and sweat glands, blood vessels and skin texture. The great majority of these changes are harmless. And the problem they present is usually a cosmetic one.

Age Spots

If you have several particularly large, dark freckles that don't fade in the winter, you have what are known as age freckles or liver spots (medically known as lentigines). Aside from their brown color, these spots have nothing at all to do with your liver. They are merely a collection of pigment cells that have increased and darkened as a result of years of exposure to the sun. Liver spots can be avoided if you take care to stay out of the sun or use sunscreens faithfully.

Numerous products on the market claim to be able to fade or eliminate age spots. But these bleaching creams aren't generally very effective.[9] They must be used twice a day for two or three months until any noticeable fading takes place. That's because fade creams don't work on the surface skin directly. They inhibit pigment cells deep below. And it takes weeks or months for these cells to work their way upward to the skin's surface. Fade creams can only lighten age spots—they do not totally eliminate them. If care is not taken to keep them on the pigmented area only, you can discolor the normal skin surrounding it.

The effect of commercial fade creams—if any—is very temporary. The spot will redarken when you stop applying the product or if you go out in the sun. Some manufacturers have begun to add sunscreen to their products to help block the sun's effects. You can always apply the sunscreen yourself, underneath the fade cream.

Physicians can prescribe more potent bleaches than those sold commercially. Or they can remove the spot through cryosurgery (a process in which the skin is frozen with liquid nitrogen) or laser surgery. A simpler alternative is to use foundation makeups to cosmetically cover the blemish.

Benign Growths

Skin tags are other blemishes which are common in the middle years. They are small, shriveled looking threads of skin that usually protrude from the armpits, breasts and sides of the neck. They are just an excess of skin and pose no health threat. But they can be easily removed, if desired.

Small, bright red bumps (called cherry angiomas) commonly form on the trunk of the body. They are caused by a collection of dilated blood vessels beneath the skin and are harmless. A physician can easily collapse such a blemish by inserting an electric needle. Also common and harmless are tiny, smooth, yellow buttonlike growths that tend to appear on the face and forehead.

Gritty, wartlike growths have a tendency to crop up on the face, neck, arms, back and hands—areas of the skin most exposed to the sun. Most such growths are benign. But it is important that you have any suspicious growth examined by a physician.

Skin Cancer

The risk of developing skin cancer increases as you age. As we've already pointed out, skin cancer is primarily caused by too much exposure to the sun. It occurs most commonly among fair-skinned people and people who spend a great deal of time outdoors. Blacks generally have a lower incidence of this type of cancer, probably because their darker pigmentation protects them from the sun.

Fortunately, skin cancers have a 90 percent cure rate, and that rate could be even higher if people were treated earlier.[10] Most forms of skin cancer do not spread to the rest of the body. One exception to this is malignant melanoma, a rare form of cancer which usually begins as a dark brown or black molelike growth that increases in size and can ulcerate and bleed. It is especially vital that this type of cancer be detected early.

You should consult a doctor whenever you notice any new or unusual skin growths or if an existing growth is changing in color or size. Seek medical care, too, if a growth itches or bleeds or a sore fails to heal. Your doctor may want to take a biopsy to make absolutely sure that the growth is not cancerous.

Removal of a growth, cancerous or otherwise, is a fairly simple procedure that can usually be done in a doctor's office. Techniques include chemical freezing or burning, scraping with a curette, surgical excision, laser surgery and the use of electric needles. Once a malignant growth is removed, the problem is usually solved. Should it grow back again, the procedure is easily repeated. Some types of malignant growths need radiation treatment.

Varicose Veins

Varicose veins tend to be hereditary. Small valves in the legs, which usually help to push blood up to the heart, fail to function. Blood pools inside the veins, and makes them become enlarged.

There is little you can do to prevent varicosities, although they can be worsened by standing for long periods of time, lack of exercise, pregnancy and sitting with legs tightly crossed. Elastic support hose and mild exercise, such as walking, may help to bring some relief, as they help the veins to pump blood back up to the heart. Women with varicose veins should take time out several times a day and elevate their legs above waist level. In severe cases, the veins may have to be surgically stripped and the branches closed off. Unfortunately, for some, the condition may reappear some years after the operation.

Don't confuse spider veins with varicose veins. Spider veins are tiny broken reddish or bluish veins beneath the skin's surface. These are also hereditary, and may become aggravated by pregnancy and sitting with your legs crossed. Spider veins are harmless. They usually disappear when injected with a salt solution.

Fat and Muscle

As you age, more of the muscle in your body is replaced by fibrous tissue. And even though you weigh about the same, you may appear heavier. Your proportions, too, may change—hips generally become less pronounced, and weight shifts to the belly and waist. All of these changes are summed up by one phrase: middle-aged spread.

While you can't completely control these events, you can slow them down. Good eating and exercise habits can keep you limber and trim. If you need confirmation of this, just look at the difference between older people who watch their weight and keep physically active, and those who sit on the sidelines with their hands in the chip dip. It's obvious that you do have a good measure of control over how well your body ages. (For a complete discussion on nutrition and exercise, see Chapters 7 and 8.)

Body Hair

After menopause you may notice an increased growth of hair on your face and body. That's because the male hormones in your bloodstream are no longer opposed by high levels of estrogen. Excess hair may appear or increase on your chin and upper lip, around your nipples or from your navel down. It's all perfectly normal, albeit cosmetically distressing.

The pattern of excess hair growth is largely determined by your genetic inheritance. Those from Southern Europe, the Middle East and Latin countries tend to have more body hair than women from Northern Europe or Scandinavia. Asian women tend to have the least body hair of all.

Since excess hair is not prized by our society, many women find this new growth pattern to be very upsetting: "The hair on my thighs has gotten so bad that I have to shave all the way up. It's a nuisance and an embarrassment. It's gotten to the point where I just don't go swimming anymore."

One fringe benefit of estrogen therapy is that it curbs the growth of body hairs. But it will not reverse the hair growth that is already present. There are, however, several effective methods for removing unwanted facial and body hairs.

Shaving

Shaving is the easiest, most convenient method of hair removal. It's recommended for legs, underarms and bikini areas. However, hair grows back rather quickly—usually within two to three days.

Many women feel that it's too masculine to shave their faces. But according to dermatologists there's nothing wrong with using this method on facial hair. One drawback, however, is that you must shave every day to avoid having stubble. A razor can give you unsightly nicks and cuts. And an electric shaver can irritate your skin.

Contrary to popular belief, shaving will not cause hair to grow in faster, thicker or darker. It cuts the hair above the skin, which is only dead tissue. The active root below is entirely unaffected. Hair may seem thicker or darker, but that's only because it's been sliced off at a blunt angle, and newly emerging hairs are more rigid and bristly. Women usually shave excess hair at a time when their hormones are changing. They may blame the increased amounts of hair on shaving, when, in fact, it would have occurred anyway.

To get the best shaving results, use a fresh razor blade (your husband's discarded razor won't do); soften stubble with warm water and shaving lather; and let the lather sit on your skin for a few minutes to further assist softening. Don't use moisturizer creams or lotions in place of shaving cream. They gunk up your razor so that it can't cut as efficiently. Use a pre-shave lotion if you are shaving with an electric shaver. It helps to dry up extra perspiration.

Instead of shaving you might want to clip facial or body hairs as close as possible to your skin surface. There are no drawbacks to clipping, except that the effects are very short-lived.

Depilatories

Depilatories are chemical creams that dissolve hair so that it can be wiped away. The hair breaks off below the surface of the skin, so results last longer (from seven to ten days), and the hairs that grow back are soft rather than stubbly. Depilatories are made for specific areas of the body: legs, arms, underarms, bikini area and upper lip. They should not be used on very delicate areas, like your breasts or upper inner thighs. A product made for one specific area of your body should never be used anywhere else.

Anything that destroys hair can also harm skin, and some people find that depilatories are irritating. They are most likely to burn your skin if they are left on longer than the time the manufacturer recommends. And they should be removed at once if any stinging or burning sensation develops.

Before you use a depilatory, it's wise to test it first on a small patch of skin. Follow the manufacturer's timing directions precisely. And check for signs of redness twenty-four hours later. If you have no skin reaction that particular product is probably safe for you to use.

Tweezing

Tweezing pulls hair out by the roots. It is good for stray facial or chest hairs, but too painful and tedious a process for larger areas. While many women tweeze their eyebrows throughout their adult lives, they may be afraid to tweeze facial hairs. There is an unfounded myth that it will cause even more hairs to sprout. While plucking in some cases can stimulate an individual hair to grow back faster, it won't cause new hairs to spread. In fact, repeated tweezing can eventually stunt hair growth.[11] Since the hair is removed by its root, it usually takes several weeks until a new hair grows back in its place.

To minimize the discomfort of tweezing, try rubbing your skin with ice before you pluck. And be sure to use a good tweezer with a firm grip—it's more apt to yank the hair out on your first try.

Waxing

In this process liquid wax is applied to the skin and allowed to set. It is then quickly whisked off along with unwanted hair. Waxing, like tweezing, pulls hair out by its roots. Its effects can last several weeks, and it's suitable for large, but less sensitive areas of skin, like the legs and arms. The procedure can be painful and, if hot wax isn't cooled sufficiently, it can cause burns. In order for this method to work the hairs must be long enough to become embedded in the wax. So a woman may have to bear with the growth of stubble in between waxings. Though home waxing kits are available, it's probably safest to have this procedure done at a reputable beauty salon.

Electrolysis

This is the only permanent method of hair removal. The hair root is destroyed after a fine needle is inserted into the hair follicle, and a weak electric current is passed through it. The procedure is uncomfortable. Since each hair root must be individually destroyed, it is slow and tedious as well. Electrolysis can be done anywhere on the body, but is most appropriate for smaller areas, like the chin and upper lip, than it is for areas with many hair follicles.

It may take months or even years of weekly sessions to completely clear an area of hair. This is due to several factors: Hair grows and falls out cyclically, so that some hairs, still beneath the surface of the skin, can be missed. About 40 to 60 percent of treated follicles are not completely destroyed, and will regenerate.[12] And brand-new hairs may continue to appear in the same spot.

It is important that electrolysis be performed by a competent and experienced operator. Improper techniques can result in scarring and pigmentation. While dermatologists rarely perform this procedure—it is just too time-consuming and costly—they may be able to refer you to someone who does. A friend who has had a satisfactory experience may be another source for referral.

Bleaches

Commercial bleaches can be used to camouflage dark hairs on your upper lip, face and body. Bleaches can be irritating, however. (They may also give very dark hair an orange cast.) So perform a twenty-four-hour patch test first, to determine whether it's safe for you to use.

Your Crowning Glory

Hair, like skin, becomes dryer around your menopausal years. The glands in your scalp may not produce as much lubricating oil. And years of perms, coloring, straightening, hair sprays, blow drying and exposure to the sun can add to the problem.

Your hair color changes too. The pigment-producing cells at the base of your hair roots shut off production. As more and more of them go on the fritz, your hair turns increasingly gray. These gray hairs are usually more wiry in texture.

Few people turn gray overnight. The process is usually a gradual one, and its timing is likely determined by heredity. Sometimes disease or poor nutrition can accelerate the rate of graying. Premature graying is usually a family trait.

Women, like men, may see their once glorious locks become painfully thin. Hair loss is common with increasing age, but it usually starts later in life for women than it does for men. And it's usually less severe. Rarely does a woman go completely bald. Instead, she may find that her hair is thinning out in the front center part of her scalp. (Underarm and pubic hair also have a tendency to become thinner with age.)

Thin and drying hair needs special consideration. To minimize loss of oils, protect it as much as possible by keeping it covered in sun, wind and extreme cold. Don't shampoo too frequently (just often enough to keep your scalp from becoming too oily). And when you do wash your hair, lather only once. Select a very mild shampoo that's formulated especially for dry hair. And always follow its use with a conditioner or cream rinse. Many beauty experts advise that you rotate shampoo and conditioning products every few weeks as the hair seems to respond better that way.

Electric hair dryers can deplete natural oils, so try not to use them excessively. If you use a blower, hold it at least six inches from your head. Exposure to a hot air dryer can be greatly reduced if you wait until your hair has partially air dried before styling it.

A weekly oil treatment can restore sheen to very dry hair. Rub some warm olive oil, mineral oil or salad oil into your scalp and hair. Wrap your hair in a towel, and let the oil penetrate for about thirty minutes, then shampoo out.

It's important to choose a good hairbrush. Nylon and natural bristles can both do the job. But you want to avoid sharp, stiff bristles that are bluntly cut. They can scratch your scalp and break your hair off. The best bristles have rounded tips and are cut in rows of varying lengths.

If thinning hair is a problem for you, choose a short, layered hairstyle. It makes hair appear thicker than it is. Unfortunately, no product has yet been found to restore scalp hair. Your best bet is to find a hairstyle which helps to camouflage the thin spots or to purchase a high-quality wig.

Chemicals in permanents, hair dyes and lacquers should be avoided when hair is already dry or brittle. And make sure you're eating a well-balanced diet. Healthy hair, like skin, is affected by what you eat.

To Dye or Not To Dye

Some women are perfectly content to let their hair go gray. They feel that it is soft and attractive. Others are upset by it. It makes them feel dowdy and drab.

If you feel unhappy about your gray hair there are many hair color alternatives available to you, including permanent dyes, temporary rinses, henna rinses and highlighting.

Permanent dyes last the longest, but are also the harshest of the coloring products so far as damage to skin and hair is concerned. In addition, there's some controversy about whether or not they can be cancer-causing.

Gaining in popularity today are the semipermanent, shampoo-in hair colors. They have a narrower color range and gradually fade out after several washings. On the other hand, they're less likely than permanent dyes to cause allergic reactions. Shampoo-in rinses can also be used to brighten gray hair and make it less yellowy.

The vegetable dye henna is made from the leaves, roots and stems of the henna plant. It has been used for coloring hair since Cleopatra's time. Because henna is a naturally derived product, it almost never irritates the skin. However, its effect on hair color is unpredictable. Some complain that it gives their hair a brassy orange color. Henna takes about five or six months to grow out. It should never be used over temporary hair rinses—the resulting mixture of colors can be quite bizarre.

Highlighting is done in a beauty salon. Strands of hair are tinted with two or three different colors, and the resulting high-low mix makes it difficult to tell when new gray hairs are growing in. Since the grays blend in so well, you can go ten to twelve weeks before you need a touch-up.

When covering gray, choose a tint that's lighter—rather than darker—than your own natural shade. Hair that's dyed too dark looks unnatural on a more mature woman. And when the gray grows back, it will be more obvious and require touch-ups more frequently. A word of caution: never use hair coloring products on lashes, eyebrows or facial hair. Always read the label: some products are not safe to use on hair that has previously been colored, straightened or permed.

To guard against an allergic reaction, conduct a patch test before you use hair coloring. Apply a small amount of the dye, tint or henna to your skin, either behind your ear or on the inside of your arm at the elbow. Leave the area uncovered for twenty-four to forty-eight hours. If redness, rashes, blisters or burning develop, you'd better not use the product. It's possible to develop a subsequent reaction to a dye that doesn't bother you at first, so manufacturers recommend that you do a preliminary patch test each and every time you color your hair.

Unpleasant color surprises can be avoided if you first try the product on a small hidden section of your hair.

Teeth

Lucky is the woman who has all of her teeth after sixty-five. Nearly half of all Americans lose most of their pearly whites by then.[13] And more women than men wear dentures after mid-life.[14] Two main causes of tooth loss have long been known: tooth decay and periodontal disease (inflamed gums and tooth sockets). But more recently, scientists are pointing an accusing finger at osteoporosis.[15]

If you want to keep flashing a nice white smile, you should watch your consumption of sweets and pay special attention to dental hygiene. The largest cause of tooth loss after forty is periodontal disease caused by plaque buildup. Plaque, a sticky, colorless film, forms on your teeth every day. It contains harmful bacteria. If it is not removed daily, it hardens into a substance called calculus, or tartar. Excessive tartar deposits may lead to inflamed and bleeding gums. Eventually, the gums become infected, tooth sockets enlarge and teeth begin to fall out.

Plaque buildup becomes more of a problem with age. According to one dental hygienist, you produce less saliva as you grow older, and saliva has a cleansing effect on the teeth. The best way to prevent periodontal disease is by daily brushing and flossing—ideally after every meal, but at the very least once a day at bedtime. Make sure your toothbrush touches all sides of the teeth, and that you pay special attention to the area where tooth meets gum. Use a toothbrush with soft bristles, and replace it every three months.

Only a dentist or dental hygienist can remove plaque once it has hardened. And it's generally recommended that you have your teeth cleaned every six months.

In some cases, postmenopausal tooth loss may be due to thinning and weakened bones rather than to plaque buildup. According to one study, women in their sixties with osteoporosis were three times as likely to have full dentures as women without the disease.[16] In light of this information, measures taken to prevent osteoporosis may also help to reduce tooth loss. (A detailed discussion of osteoporosis is presented in Chapter 11.)

If you smoke cigarettes, you increase your chances of getting periodontal disease as well as osteoporosis. The link between cigarette smoking and tooth loss has been well documented.[17]

Eyes

The eyes are not exempt from the aging process. Young eyes have soft, flexible lenses, made of gel-like material. As we reach forty, the gel begins to harden and the eye loses its ability to focus on nearby objects. The condition is known as presbyopia. And if you have to hold print at arm's length in order to read it, it's a sure bet that you've got it. (Tired eyes or headaches while doing close work are other symptoms.) There's no way to stop or reverse these natural changes in lens structure. But glasses, contact lenses or bifocals help to restore close-up vision. You may find that you need a new prescription every two years or so, as the lens continues to harden. Your vision should level off by the time you are sixty.[18]

Floaters may also become noticeable once you are past thirty-five. They're small black specks or "wiggles" that you may see when you look at a light background, like the sky. Floaters are created when the gel-like fluid on the inner part of the eye separates and becomes stringy. Sometimes the floaters fade and disappear. They are not harmful. However, if you suddenly see a lot of dark spots, you may have a more serious condition and should consult an opthalmologist.

Another condition that might develop as you grow older is cataracts. Cataracts are hazy spots that form on all or part of the lens and block out the passage of light. Cataracts occur most often in people over forty—especially if there is a family history of the disease. Symptoms include blurred and fuzzy vision, "ghost" images and an increased sensitivity to light. Most cataracts develop slowly, over many years. Others occur more quickly. If the cataract doesn't seriously impair vision it may not be necessary to remove it. However, if it interferes with daily activities, like sewing, reading or driving, surgery may be recommended, and the entire lens will be removed. After the operation, the eye can no longer focus on its own. Special eyeglasses or contact lenses will have to be prescribed; or the doctor can insert a permanent plastic lens directly into the eye during surgery.

Glaucoma, one of the leading causes of blindness, affects two out of every one hundred people—most over thirty-five years of age.[19] It is a buildup of pressure inside the eye that can eventually destroy the optic nerve. Glaucoma is insidious in that it gives little warning. By the time a person notices any loss of sight, it's too late to undo the damage. Glaucoma can be easily detected in its early stages by a simple, painless test. When discovered early, loss of sight can be slowed or prevented with eyedrops, medication, laser treatments and, if need be, surgery. Symptoms of optic nerve damage may include a loss of side vision, blurred or foggy vision and an inability for eyes to adjust to a darkened room. While treatments will stop further progress of the disease, they cannot restore vision that has already been impaired.

If you are a diabetic, and have had the disease for fifteen or more years, you are more likely than the average middle-aged person to develop diabetic retinopathy—leaking blood vessels at the back of the eye.[20] This condition can eventually lead to blindness. It can be treated by laser lights that seal the leaking blood vessels. All diabetics should be sure to visit their opthalmologist regularly.

After menopause, when mucous membranes become thinner and glands less active, some people suffer from dry eyes. In this condition, tear glands produce too few tears, and the eyes itch and burn. Eyedrop solutions, called "artificial tears," must be applied frequently to keep the eye moist.

Eyesight is too precious a commodity to take chances with. Beginning at age thirty-five, you should have a full eye exam, including a check for glaucoma, every two to three years. The person best equipped to diagnose and treat eye disorders is an eye doctor, or ophthalmologist.

Fighting Back

"Why fight aging?" asks one woman. "It's not really so bad when you consider the alternative." A droll observation—but a true one. Everyone must accept certain inevitable physical changes that come with aging. But that doesn't mean you should take them lying down. In fact, it would be better to walk, jog or swim well into your later years. Eyes, hair, skin, teeth . . . all need special attention to remain healthy and attractive as you age. That means giving your body extra t.l.c., eating nutritious foods and applying principles of preventive health care to your daily life. While nothing can stop the passage of years, you can continue to look and feel your best at any age.

Chapter 11
Osteoporosis

"I think it all started twenty years ago, although I didn't know it at the time. I had aches and pains in my spine and joints and was diagnosed as having arthritis. I wasn't told anything about needing extra calcium or estrogen. Nothing was mentioned about osteoporosis. I took prednisone for many years. It was the only thing that made the pain bearable. Only within the last few years have I discovered that prednisone is a bone thinner, and that you're not supposed to be on it as long as I was.

"Over the years my spine became very curved. I had terrible pains and was in and out of the hospital. My X rays showed that I had multiple spinal fractures. 'That can't be possible,' I told the doctor. 'I didn't have any accidental falls.' That's when it was explained to me that I had osteoporosis. My bones had become so thin that they fractured by themselves.

"Within the last two years I lost seven inches of height—

I'm now only four feet seven inches tall. I'm in constant pain, mainly in my shoulder blades, collarbone and lower back. I used to like to dance. Now I have trouble even walking to the corner. I can't stand straight. I can't bend. I'm so hunched over that I can't even reach to the shelves to get the dishes. If I exert myself just the least, I get terribly short of breath. My husband has to help me with everything.

"I'm now taking calcium pills and estrogen. I wish I knew more about these things when I was younger. Maybe my condition wouldn't have progressed to this point. Now it's too late. I'm told I just have to live with it."—Age seventy-four.

"My mother is seventy-two years old and has lost three inches of height. She gets backaches, but the doctor says it's from her arthritis. Though she's a little stooped over, she doesn't look too bad, and she's able to drive and get around all right. My mother's mother really shrunk down in size as she got older. The curvature of her back was much more noticeable. She used to make jokes about it and say that we grandchildren were almost as tall as she was. Do you think my mother could have osteoporosis? And that my grandmother had it too? I have to admit, I really don't know too much about it."—Age forty.

Osteoporosis means porous bones. It's a condition in which the bones become so thin that they can no longer support the skeletal structure. In severe cases a minor fall, or ordinary lifting movement (like picking up a bag of groceries), or even a strong sneeze, may result in serious fractures. One of four American women over the age of sixty is affected by this disease. Each year it is responsible for an estimated 700,000 fractures.[1] As the population in this country ages, osteoporosis is becoming a more widespread problem.

A Woman's Disease

Your skeleton appears to be a hard, white, permanent structure. But it is actually composed of living tissue and blood vessels. Throughout your life, bone is constantly being broken down and absorbed by your body, and then built up again in a process called remodeling.

Bone, like any other living tissue, is affected by aging. As people grow older their bones do not repair themselves as quickly as they used to. Beginning at about age thirty-five both men and women lose a little more bone than is formed. This is the start of a slow but gradual loss of skeletal mass, which is considered to be a normal part of aging for both sexes.

Women lose bone at the normal rate until they reach menopause. Here the sexes part company. Declining estrogen levels seem to hasten the breakdown of bone. In the five or six years following menopause women lose bone twice as quickly as men of comparable age.[2] It is not unusual for a woman to have a 1 to 2 percent bone loss per year, and to eventually wind up with 30 to 50 percent less skeletal mass by the time she reaches age seventy-five. (Men, on the other hand, rarely lose more than 15 to 20 percent of their bone mass by old age.) The rate of bone loss among menopausal women gradually decreases, and by age sixty-five becomes equal again to a man's.[3,4,5,6]

This is not to say that men don't get osteoporosis too. But the incidence among men is far lower (eight times more women have it), and it usually becomes apparent later in life and is generally less severe.[7]

Men have several protective advantages not shared by females. The male hormone testosterone appears to have a bone-preserving effect for men much the same as estrogen does for women. But men have a very gradual decline in testosterone levels—nothing like the rapid hormonal fluctuations a woman experiences at menopause. In addition, men generally have heavier, denser bones than women. So a loss of bone with age doesn't take as heavy a toll.

Male exercise and diet patterns also tend to bolster the growth of bone. Men are usually more physically active and do more heavy work than women—and this increased physical activity helps to build bone mass. Because they generally eat more, men are likely to consume more of the bone-building mineral, calcium. They are also less apt than women to go on repeated weight-loss diets that restrict calcium intake.

Women with poor eating habits face the additional risk of losing calcium from their bones during pregnancy and lactation. And, since older bones are thinner bones, a woman's superior longevity also increases her risk of fractures.

How Osteoporosis Progresses

Osteoporosis is often referred to as a silent disease. The bones thin out slowly over the years without any outward sign. In most cases a bone fracture is the first clue that a woman has this condition. But by this time, osteoporosis has already caused irreversible damage.

Each bone in your body consists of a solid outer layer (cortical bone); and a porous, honeycomb-like inner material (trabecular bone). The porous trabecular bone is the first to feel the effects of osteoporosis. The holes within it widen like Swiss cheese, until it is eventually unable to support the surrounding cortical shell. Although osteoporotic bone has the same chemical composition as normal bone, it is thinner and much more fragile. A slight fall or blow is all that is needed to fracture it.

The bones in the spinal column (vertebrae) are usually the first to become injured by osteoporosis. That's because they are made largely of trabecular bone. Spinal vertebrae may fracture and collapse spontaneously, or after a simple stretching movement, like making the bed or lifting a child. One out

Normal Bone   Osteoporotic bone

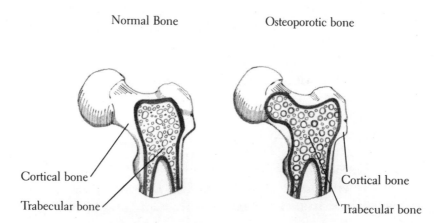

Cortical bone   Cortical bone

Trabecular bone   Trabecular bone

of four women has at least one vertebral fracture by the age of sixty; by age seventy-five, that number jumps to one out of two.[8]

Some people have backaches and muscle spasms after a vertebra collapses. The pain may last weeks or months and then completely subside. But many women never have any pain at all. In fact, vertebral fractures are often discovered during X-ray exams for unrelated disorders.

The term "little old lady" aptly describes the victim of repeated spinal fractures. Every time a vertebra collapses, a woman loses about an inch of height. It is possible to lose several inches within a span of several weeks. In very severe cases, some women become as much as eight inches shorter. That means a 5'5" woman could end up being 4'9".

Since the leg bones aren't affected, a woman loses all of her height from her waist up. If many of her vertebrae have caved in, her spinal column will form an exaggerated curve, her rib cage will fall, and her stomach will protrude. This condition is popularly known as the "dowager's hump." It is the cause of severe, chronic back pain, as well as digestive and breathing difficulties. The physical deformity also exacts a psychological toll. A woman's appearance is changed forever, and her normal activities are greatly restricted.

Wrist fractures are a common early sign of osteoporosis. They typically occur when a woman puts out her hand to stop a fall. Fractures of the wrist are ten times more common among women in their fifties than they are among men.[9] They usually heal within weeks and cause no long-term effects. However, if you fracture your wrist after a relatively minor impact, you'd do well to consider this an early warning sign of osteoporosis. Preventive measures taken now may help to minimize future bone loss.

Periodontal disease is another possible warning sign. Osteoporosis thins out the jawbone, so that teeth eventually loosen and fall out. Because the jawbone continues to shrink, it is often very difficult to get dentures to fit properly. Sometimes a dentist can spot early osteoporosis from evidence of jawbone loss on dental X rays.

Hip fractures are by far the most serious consequence of osteoporosis. Since hip bones are made largely of cortical

Progressive Height Loss

As more and more vertebrae weaken and collapse a woman's spine becomes curved and she can lose up to 8" in height. All height is lost from the waist up.

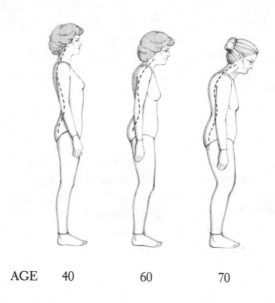

AGE   40   60   70

bone, they don't fracture until relatively late in life, when osteoporosis is in a very advanced state. Some 200,000 such injuries per year are attributed to osteoporosis, at a medical cost of over one billion dollars. Half of the victims never recover their full mobility, and many must have ancillary home care or be placed in nursing homes. Hip fractures are the twelfth leading cause of death in the United States: nearly 20 percent of those afflicted die within three months from complications—including pneumonia and blood clots—due to prolonged bed confinement. Hip fractures are most often the result of a fall, but it's possible for the hip bone to become so thin that it fractures spontaneously and causes a fall. If a woman fractures one hip she has a twenty times greater risk of fracturing the other hip as well.[10,11,12,13]

High-Risk Factors

It's impossible to predict ahead of time who will get osteoporosis and who will not. However, there are some factors that may put a woman at greater risk for getting this disease.

Age

The older you are, the thinner your bones will probably be. Barring disease or congenital abnormalities, osteoporosis is rarely seen in young people. That's because bone becomes progressively thinner with age. In addition, older people have greater difficulty absorbing and utilizing calcium, particularly once over sixty.

Menopause

After menopause, declining estrogen levels seem to step up bone loss. Scientists aren't sure exactly how estrogen affects the bones. Bones don't contain any estrogen receptors, and are not affected directly by this hormone the way the uterus and breasts are. Perhaps estrogen influences other hormones, signaling them to form or destroy the bones. For whatever reason, high estrogen levels do keep the skeleton from losing mass.

The earlier in life that estrogen levels fall, the higher the risk of osteoporosis. This is one of the reasons why it's best for the ovaries to remain intact when a premenopausal woman undergoes a hysterectomy. Women with a normal menopause have a 25 percent risk of osteoporosis; those with a premature menopause, or whose ovaries are removed or destroyed before the age of forty-five, have a 50 percent risk of this disease. Women who are still menstruating after fifty lose bone at a slower rate than menopausal women of the same age.[14,15]

Heredity

Osteoporosis runs in families: if your mother, sister, grandmother or aunt had osteoporosis, your chances of getting it are higher than if there were no family history of the disease.

Whether or not you get osteoporosis is partly determined by your racial inheritance. Rates are highest among Chinese,

Japanese and Caucasians from Northern Europe and the British Isles. The lowest incidence is found among blacks, Hispanics and those of Mediterranean ancestry. Jewish women seem to fall somewhere in the middle range.[16]

As a group, some races may lose bone at higher rates than others. And some populations are endowed with bigger, stronger skeletal structures which are less vulnerable to fractures. Black men, for example, have the highest bone mass of all and are relatively immune from osteoporosis. Black women and white men have an intermediate amount of bone and a low incidence of this disease. White and Asian women have the least amount of bone and are the prime candidates for fractures.

Skin pigmentation seems to be another predictor of bone loss. Among white women, those with red or blond hair and very fair complexions are usually most prone to osteoporosis.

Body Size

Short, slender, delicately boned white women are at higher risk for osteoporosis. They have less bone to lose before their skeletons become easily fractured. Obese women are at lower risk for the disease. The stress of the excess weight on their skeletons stimulates their bones to grow bigger. And since a woman's fat cells help to manufacture estrogen after menopause, an obese woman has higher postmenopausal estrogen levels.

Exercise

As people grow older they tend to be less active. Unfortunately, inactivity can contribute to loss of bone mass. In extreme cases, people who are bedridden or whose limbs are broken or paralyzed, suffer from severe and rapid loss of bone—sometimes within a matter of weeks. Astronauts, though active in space, rapidly lose bone due to conditions of weightlessness. Exercise, on the other hand, can actually increase bone mass. Athletes have stronger, thicker bones than nonathletes. And tennis players have more bone density in their playing arms. Studies of postmenopausal women in nursing homes have shown that light to moderate exercise

Osteoporosis Checklist
Are You At Risk?

The following risk factors may make you a likely candidate for osteoporosis.

( ) Caucasian or Asian.
( ) Past menopause.
( ) Small-boned.
( ) Slender.
( ) Fair-complexioned.
( ) Family history of the disease (mother, sister, aunt).
( ) Low calcium intake
( ) High amounts of dietary protein (especially from red meat).
( ) Sedentary lifestyle.
( ) Heavy smoker.
( ) Heavy drinker.
( ) No children.
( ) Early menopause (either naturally or from surgical removal of the ovaries).
( ) Chronic stress or illness.
( ) Chronic dieting.

can slow bone loss and in some cases even increase new bone formation.[17]

Calcium

Inadequate calcium intake is considered a very important factor in the development of osteoporosis. If you have eaten ample amounts of calcium throughout your childhood and adult life, you reach menopause with denser bones. And the denser the bones, the more protection you have against fractures later on. Studies of both people and laboratory animals have shown a link between osteoporosis and calcium-deficient diets.[18]

The calcium in your bones is like money in the bank. While 99 percent of the calcium is concentrated in your skeleton, to give it strength and structure, the other 1 percent is in your blood. The circulating calcium helps regulate some vital body processes, including normal heart beat, nerve conduction, muscle contraction and enzyme activation. Each day some of this calcium leaves your body—through perspiration, feces and urine. If you fail to replenish it by eating a calcium-rich diet, your body goes to its calcium bank, and withdraws the mineral from your bones. You then create what's known as a negative calcium balance. If this goes on for too many years, your bones become weak and thin.

Calcium is a relatively plentiful nutrient, available in many foods. Yet, on any given day, over three-quarters of American women over thirty-five fall far short of the 800 mg. Recommended Dietary Allowance.[19,20] In fact, most women in this age group take in only 450 mg. of calcium a day. This translates into an average bone loss of 1.5 percent per year.[21]

After menopause your need for calcium increases—both because you lose bone at a greater rate, and because your body's ability to absorb calcium declines with age. It's ironic that so many women cut down on this nutrient at the time they require it the most.

Dietary Imbalances

Too little or too much of some foods may tip your calcium balance in the wrong direction and increase your chances of osteoporosis. Diets that are heavy in protein (from too much red meat) may cause you to lose more calcium in your urine. An excessive amount of fiber (usually not a problem in this country) can hamper calcium absorption. So can too much phosphorous (found in soda, processed foods and red meats) and salt. Several studies have shown that vegetarians have stronger, denser skeletons than meat eaters. They also lose bone at a slower rate and develop osteoporosis less frequently.[22] This may be because meat contains high amounts of phosphorous. Meat also creates an acid balance in your body which may add to the breakdown of bone.

Vitamin D is necessary for calcium absorption, and a deficiency can raise the risks of osteoporosis. This vitamin is easily obtained by most people—through vitamin-fortified dairy products, fish oils, egg yolks and sunshine. And deficiencies are rare. Elderly people who are confined indoors, and who do not eat properly, however, may not get enough of this vitamin.

Diseases

Certain diseases and conditions seem to predispose an individual to osteoporosis. These include rheumatoid arthritis, chronic kidney disease and disorders of the thyroid, parathyroid or adrenal glands. Those who have part of their stomach surgically removed, as a result of cancer or ulcers, are also at higher risk.[23]

Drugs

Among drugs that increase bone loss and lead to a higher risk of osteoporosis are: thyroid replacement drugs; heparin (an anticoagulant); cortisone preparations (such as prednisone); aluminum-containing antacids; anticonvulsants; and the antibiotic drug tetracycline.[24,25,26] Some diuretics increase loss of calcium through the urine, while others (notably thiazide diuretics) may actually have a positive effect on bone.[27] Excessive amounts of caffeine in the diet impair calcium absorption. So does too much alcohol. Alcoholics tend to have a smaller bone mass than nondrinkers. They also have a decreased appetite and are likely to drink in place of eating nutritious foods.

Oral contraceptive users may have an edge when it comes to osteoporosis. Long-term pill users are likely to have stronger bones.[28]

Smoking

Smokers have a higher risk of osteoporosis, especially if they are slender. There are several possible explanations for this. Heavy smokers experience menopause about five years earlier than nonsmokers, and the earlier the menopause, the greater the bone loss.[29] Smoking may also interfere with vitamin absorption and bone metabolism. In addition, smokers usually weigh less; this too contributes to the risk of losing bone.

Pregnancy

Childbearing may have a protective effect on the bones, providing the expectant mother is well nourished. Pregnancy increases levels of progesterone and estrogen—and appears to stimulate new bone formation. When a pregnant woman fails to take in enough calcium, however, just the opposite can be true. The baby's calcium supply will come from the mother's bones, thus increasing the risk of osteoporosis in later years. Breastfeeding, too, can deplete a woman's calcium reserves if she is not properly nourished. Women who have never borne children appear to be at greater risk for osteoporosis than those who have.

Stress

Prolonged periods of emotional stress, grief, boredom, illness or anxiety can deplete your body's calcium reserves and expose you to bone loss.

Diagnosing Osteoporosis

It's very difficult to diagnose osteoporosis in its early stages. By the time a woman feels pain or has an obvious fracture, much of her bone mass has already been lost. Scientists need a fast, easy, inexpensive way of screening the general population. The ideal would be a technique that could periodically measure a woman's bone mass. Then fast bone losers could be singled out and given appropriate treatment.

Conventional X rays have not been found to be very useful. Over 30 percent of a woman's bone mass must be lost before it can be detected on X-ray film. Computerized tomography (CAT scan) is more sensitive to the loss of small amounts of bone, but the procedure exposes a woman to large amounts of radiation and is extremely costly.

More promising is the development of a relatively new technique called photon absorptiometry. A machine called a bone densitometer is used to measure the thickness, width and mineral content of the bones by calculating how many gamma rays the bones absorb. The machine emits a fraction of the radiation of conventional X rays and is sensitive enough to detect a bone loss of from 1 to 3 percent.[30] There are two types of photon absorptiometry: single photon absorptiometry, a ten-minute procedure which can measure bone loss in a woman's forearm; and dual photon absorptiometry, which takes up to an hour, but can determine the amount of bone mineral lost anywhere in the entire skeleton.

Bone densitometers are very sophisticated and expensive machines. They are currently being used mainly in research centers, and are unavailable to most physicians. However, their importance in the early detection of osteoporosis is becoming more apparent. And it is likely that they will be made more widely available in the years to come.

Work is also being done on the development of a diagnostic blood test that could be performed in a doctor's office.[31] To date, however, no accurate blood or urine analyses for osteoporosis have yet been devised.

If you think you're at high risk for osteoporosis, you might contact the orthopedics department at a local teaching hospital, or call your county medical association and ask if there are any bone densitometers being used in your area.

You should also be alert for signs that you are losing height. Have your doctor measure you at your annual visits, or measure yourself periodically at home. To determine your height, remove your shoes and stand with your back against the wall. Your head should be upright, your knees straight and your heels together. Another, though less accurate way to gauge whether or not you have lost height is to compare the width of your arm span to your present height. In the normal, mature adult the two measurements should be about the same.

Preventive Measures

Once bone mass is lost, there is little you can do to restore it. So the best approach to osteoporosis is a preventive one. The object is to help make your bones as dense as possible before menopause. The thicker your skeleton at menopause, the more margin you have for bone loss.

The following are preventive measures which are generally recommended by medical authorities:

1. *Eat a calcium-rich diet.* Calcium is important throughout a woman's lifetime. Although bones no longer grow in

size from ages eighteen to thirty-five, they do continue to become increasingly dense. If a woman eats enough calcium during these years, she can build her bones up to their maximum potential. They are then less likely to fracture after menopause. The Recommended Dietary Allowance of calcium for adults is 800 mg. After normal bone loss begins—at about age thirty-five to forty—calcium intake must be stepped up further. It is generally recommended that women over forty consume at least 1,000 mg. per day, and that women past menopause take in 1,200 to 1,500 mg. daily.[32] Postmenopausal women taking oral estrogen need about 1,000 mg. of calcium daily.[33]

The best source of calcium is dairy products. Milk contains other nutrients—like vitamin D, phosphorous and lactose—in just the proportions that help your body absorb calcium most efficiently. Calcium supplements are also available, and a woman may want to supplement a low-calcium diet with 500 to 1000 mg. daily in order to bring her intake up to the recommended totals. (A complete discussion on calcium-containing foods and supplements appears in Chapter 7.)

Your need for calcium may increase when you are ill or emotionally stressed, and if you are dieting. Try to have extra servings of calcium-containing foods, or to take calcium supplements at such times. If stress becomes a chronic problem you may find it helpful to practice stress reduction techniques, as discussed in Chapter 5.

2. *Avoid dietary excesses.* Protein can hamper calcium absorption. So if you are a big meat eater, consider incorporating some vegetarian dishes into your weekly menu. The adult requirement for protein is 44 gm. a day, or the equivalent of 6 oz. of meat. Red meat, with its high phosphorous content, shouldn't be eaten more than a few times a week (substitute fish and poultry in its place). Avoid also the over-liberal use of salt. You get more than enough of your daily sodium quota in the foods that you eat.

Most Americans eat too little—rather than too much—fiber. But if you're in the latter category, remember fibrous foods, too, can reduce calcium absorption. High-fiber foods and calcium-containing foods probably shouldn't be eaten at the same sitting.

Megadoses of vitamins should also be avoided. While vitamin D is essential to the proper absorption of calcium, too much can actually cause bones to thin out. The average adult requires approximately 400 IU of vitamin D daily, an amount which can easily be obtained through fortified dairy products and exposure to the sun. Vitamin A in excess is also known to decrease bone content.

Can too much calcium supplementation be harmful? Some fear that it may cause kidney stones. Authorities generally believe that up to 2,000 mg. a day can safely be consumed without any ill effects (this takes into account the calcium from your diet as well as from supplements).[34] However, if you have a personal or family history of kidney stones you should not take calcium supplements without your doctor's okay. When taking calcium supplements make sure to drink plenty of fluids each day.

3. *Exercise daily.* This is the only preventive measure that can actually add mass to bones, provided a woman is also getting sufficient calcium. Bones, like muscles, get bigger when added stress is placed on them. Exercise also improves circulation, bringing more bone-building nutrients to the skeleton. The most effective bone-building exercises are those which stress the long bones of the body (arms and legs). These include jogging, walking, hiking, bicycling, aerobics and rope jumping. While swimming is a good all-around body conditioner, it does not put enough stress on the bones to build them up. For a complete discussion of how to start an exercise program, see Chapter 8.

Overly strenuous exercise can be as bad for your bones as no exercise at all. Women athletes and ballet dancers who stop menstruating as a result of exercise may put themselves at greater risk for bone loss. In one study, women runners who no longer had periods had 28 percent less bone mass than a matched control group. It is believed that low amounts of body fat among female athletes reduce their estrogen levels, which contributes to early bone loss.[35]

4. *Avoid substances that interfere with calcium absorption.* Both smoking and drinking can rob your bones of calcium. How much of these substances are too much? There are, as yet, no satisfactory guidelines. The chances of osteoporosis

rise with the number of cigarettes smoked, however.[36] And chronic alcoholics are known to have thinner bones at every age.[37] If you don't eliminate these substances from your life, at least cut back. And be extra vigilant about your calcium intake.

Should you be on a medication that's known to cause bone thinning, ask your doctor about the possibility of switching to another type of drug, or about the advisability of taking calcium supplements.

5. *Consider estrogen therapy if you are high risk.* Estrogen therapy has been proven in many studies to prevent or greatly reduce bone loss after menopause. Its long-term use can reduce the incidence of spine, wrist and hip fractures by 60 to 70 percent.[38] In order to be most effective, the hormone must be administered within the first three years of menopause— before any significant bone loss occurs.

Since estrogen therapy does entail possible risks, its use among healthy women remains controversial. (See Chapter 6 for a complete discussion of the pros and cons of estrogen therapy.) One gynecologist, who believes in giving estrogen across the board, puts it this way: "Painful intercourse, hot flashes and vaginal atrophy are not likely to kill. Osteoporosis is potentially fatal. I don't want my women patients dying of it. I lean toward exercise, calcium and estrogen as preventives." Judy Norsigian, a founder of The Boston Women's Health Book Collective, expresses the opposite viewpoint: "Yes, 25 percent of all women get osteoporosis, but the other 75 percent don't. Why should women be taking hormones that they may not need to be taking and that may be associated with problems?"

Most experts do agree that hormone treatment is important for women with premature menopause, either naturally or surgically, since this group is at very high risk of osteoporosis. Other women who might be considered candidates for estrogen therapy are thin, small-boned Caucasians with a poor calcium intake and a family history of the disease.

It is unclear how long a woman must stay on estrogen in order for it to be effective against bone loss. Present studies span only about a decade, but studies of twenty to thirty years have to be conducted before a final conclusion can be drawn.

In one study, the benefits of estrogen were rapidly lost once therapy was discontinued.[39] It seems as if estrogen therapy must be long-term in order to keep bone from losing mass.

The addition of progesterone to estrogen therapy doesn't seem to have any harmful effects on bone mass. In fact, several studies have shown that this hormone may even promote bone formation.[40]

Treatments for Osteoporosis

Once a woman has osteoporosis, there is little that can be done to restore bone to normal. Treatment is aimed at preventing further bone loss, and includes combinations of estrogen therapy and calcium supplements (to reduce bone loss) and vitamin D (to increase calcium absorption). Estrogen is not as effective in halting bone loss when given more than six years after menopause. Vitamin D is toxic in large amounts and supplements should be taken only under a doctor's supervision.

The use of sodium fluoride to treat osteoporosis is controversial. Fluoride encourages calcium retention and is also believed to harden bones. It has been added to the water supply systems in many areas in order to prevent tooth decay. Two studies suggest that people living in areas with high levels of naturally occurring fluoride in their drinking water have a lower incidence of osteoporosis, although another study refutes this claim.[41]

Fluoride is very promising because it can actually stimulate formation of new bone. However, high doses can result in severe side effects, such as gastrointestinal bleeding, stomach pain and nausea, as well as swollen and painful joints. Not enough is yet known about safe dosage levels or possible long-term effects. Another drawback is that fluoride-stimulated bone tends to be more crystalline, therefore more easily fractured than normal bone.[42]

Ongoing research is being done on other hormones that may help to control osteoporosis. These include parathyroid hormone, calcitonin, and stanozolol, a male hormone. Thiazide diuretics, usually given to control high blood pressure or swelling, have been shown to reduce calcium loss, and may prove helpful in treating osteoporosis.[43]

Since physical inactivity leads to more bone loss, exercise among osteoporotic women is encouraged whenever possible. Jogging or other strenuous activities might cause another fracture. But walking, and mild forms of muscle-strengthening exercise may be performed under a doctor's guidance. Although swimming is not generally recommended as a bone-building exercise, it places little stress on the body, and may be suitable for women who have more advanced cases of the disease.

It's important not to place undue stress on an already weakened spine. Whether you suffer from osteoporosis or not, it's good to practice proper body mechanics. Learn to carry heavy things close to your body. When picking objects up, never bend from the waist. Instead, bend your knees and lower yourself gently into a squatting position. As you lift, keep your back straight and your knees apart.

The Future Looks Brighter

More breakthroughs in osteoporosis have been made in this decade than in all years past. With sophisticated machinery and new technologies, it may soon be possible to detect and halt bone loss in its very early stages. In the meantime, it is within every woman's power to take some simple bone-saving measures: make sure you get enough calcium every day; exercise regularly; and consult your doctor about hormone therapy if you fall into the high-risk category. Perhaps one day there will be a way to restore bone after it is lost. In the meantime, prevention holds the key to your future health.

Chapter 12
Staying Healthy:
A Gynecologic
Guide

As you approach menopause, you are at greater risk for a number of gynecologic diseases. Cancers of the breast, uterus and ovaries are seen most often in women past forty. In most cases, early detection results in a more favorable outcome, so it is especially important that you practice good preventive health care. This should include an annual gynecologic checkup.

Your yearly gynecologic exam may be performed by a gynecologist, internist, general practitioner or family practitioner. In a growing number of medical practices, nurse-practitioners do well-care exams and give medical counseling.

An office visit should provide an opportunity for you to ask questions and learn something about your body. If you have any special concerns, write them down on a notepad beforehand and bring it along with you. Your health care provider should set aside ample time in which to sit down and talk with you. If you feel that your treatment is consistently rushed or impersonal, you might consider shopping around for another physician. Communication between patient and physician is more than a courtesy. It is an important part of good medical care.

The Annual Exam

Your health care provider will want to begin the exam with a detailed personal and family medical history. A thorough physical exam includes the following:

• An examination of nose, throat, eyes and thyroid gland.
• Blood pressure and weight measurements.
• Routine blood and urine checks.
• A heart and lung check with a stethoscope.
• Palpation of your abdomen and back to check for enlargement or swelling of liver, spleen and kidneys.
• Breast and pelvic exams.
• A Pap test.
• A rectal exam.

You might also ask your doctor to keep a record of your height, so that you have some idea of how much bone you lose after menopause. (See Chapter 11: Osteoporosis.)

The Pelvic Exam

External Exam

The pelvic exam begins with an examination of your external genital area. Your physician will examine your labia and clitoris to make sure that there are no signs of infection, such as irritation, swelling or redness.

Speculum Exam

A metal or plastic instrument, called a speculum, is then inserted and opened within your vagina to spread your vaginal walls apart. (A metal speculum can be uncomfortably cold, and some physicians will warm it before insertion.) The speculum permits the physician to examine your vaginal lining, as well as your cervix, for lesions, irritations, unusual discharges or growths. Some practitioners keep a mirror handy to permit a woman to see her cervix during the exam. This view from the other side of the stirrups is one a woman doesn't often get to see.

You may feel some pressure upon insertion of the speculum, but there should not be any pain. If there is, tell your health care provider. He or she may be able to reposition the speculum or use one that's a smaller size.

Pap Smear

The Pap smear is done while the speculum is still in place. A cotton swab or wooden or plastic spatula is used to scrape a thin layer of cells from your cervix. The cervical tissue is

Pelvic Exam and Pap Smear

The speculum is used to spread your vaginal walls apart to permit a better view of the cervix. Then a wooden spatula or cotton swab scrapes away some cervical cells for laboratory analysis.

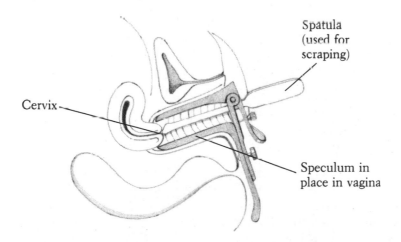

Spatula (used for scraping)

Cervix

Speculum in place in vagina

then smeared on a glass slide, "fixed" with a chemical and sent to a lab for evaluation. The main purpose of the Pap smear is to detect cervical cancer. It does so with a 95 percent rate of accuracy.[1] The Pap smear cannot reliably detect uterine or ovarian cancers: it does so with only 15 to 50 percent accuracy.[2]

There is some medical disagreement over how often a woman should have a Pap smear. The American Cancer Society says that after two initial normal smears, one year apart, you need only have a Pap smear once every three years. Their recommendation is based on cost-effectiveness studies and on the fact that cervical cancers are usually very slow growing.[3] The American College of Obstetricians and Gynecologists strongly disagrees. A small percentage of cervical cancers are fast-growing, they assert, and a yearly Pap test is the best means of early detection.[4] Ask your doctor his or her opinion on this matter. Since a Pap smear involves no risk to you, it would seem more sensible to err on the side of safety and have one annually. This is especially true if you are at high risk for cervical cancer. (Risk factors include early age at first intercourse, multiple sex partners and many pregnancies.)

There are several classification systems currently used to interpret Pap smear results. The oldest and most commonly used classification system divides results into five categories: Class I: Normal cells. Class II: Abnormal infection cells. Class III: Mild precancerous changes. Class IV: Severe precancerous changes. Class V: True cervical cancer.

Cervical cancers progress very slowly, so if you have routine Pap smears, your chances of catching the condition in its early stages are excellent. When detected early, cervical cancer is effectively treated nearly 100 percent of the time.[5]

Abnormal Pap smears are common and do not necessarily mean that a woman has cancer. They frequently revert to normal when repeated within a few months. The most typical reason for an abnormal Pap smear is the presence of a cervical or vaginal infection. Sometimes abnormal cells are removed by burning (cautery) or freezing (cryosurgery). Most recently, laser surgery is being used for this purpose. Should cancer be diagnosed, it must be confirmed by a subsequent biopsy.

The Bimanual Exam

The practitioner feels the size, shape and consistency of your pelvic organs.

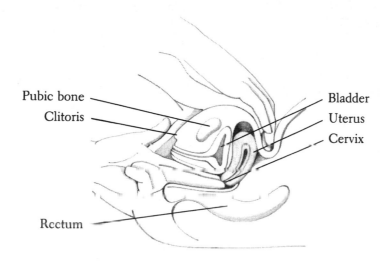

Pubic bone

Clitoris

Bladder

Uterus

Cervix

Rectum

The Bimanual Exam

The second part of an internal exam is called a bimanual (both hands) exam. The physician inserts two gloved fingers of one hand into your vagina, and presses with the other hand on various areas of your lower abdomen. This permits the practitioner to tell the size, consistency and shape of your ovaries, uterus and fallopian tubes, whether or not they are swollen or tender, or if any abnormal growths are present. Some women may feel a twinge when their ovaries are examined.

The Rectal Exam

With the index finger in the vagina and the middle finger in the rectum, the physician can feel the position and tone of the pelvic organs, and may also check the rectum for any masses or lesions.

Pelvic exams should not be painful. When you relax your abdominal muscles you decrease your discomfort and help your practitioner to more easily feel your pelvic organs. Many women find it helpful to do deep breathing during the internal exam, focusing on the rhythm of their breath or on a picture or object in the examining room.

Breast Self-Examination

Breast cancer is the leading cause of death in women ages thirty-seven to fifty-five.[6] One of eleven women each year will contract this disease. And an estimated 38,400 will die from it.[7] It is thought that those at higher than average risk are women over fifty, those whose sisters or mothers had the disease (especially before menopause), and those who have already had a breast lump themselves. There is a possible link between breast cancer and diets high in fat. However, this has not been conclusively proven.

For many years it was believed that breast cancer always spread in an orderly fashion—from the breast to the lymph nodes to the rest of the body. Now it seems that, in some forms, the cancer is already present in the rest of the body before it can be detected in the breast.[8,9]

Scientists don't yet know the causes of breast cancer. And, unfortunately, it seems as though little can be done to prevent it. However, the prognosis is best when the disease is caught in its earliest stages.

Though an annual medical breast exam is helpful in breast cancer detection, monthly breast self-examinations can be more valuable. You are in the best position to know the normal feel and texture of your own breasts and to detect any changes from month to month. Eighty or 90 percent of all breast lumps are found by women themselves or by their partners.[10,11]

Many women resist learning breast self-examination. They feel that it is best left to doctors who know the proper technique. Breast self-examination is not very difficult to master, and it takes only minutes to do. Ask your health care provider to demonstrate the technique to you at your annual exam.

Then try doing it yourself. Your practitioner will be able to tell you if you are doing it correctly.

The specter of losing a breast to cancer is so horrifying that some women can't get themselves to feel for lumps; others delay seeking treatment once a lump is found. "I know it's irrational," says a thirty-eight year old, "but I'm so frightened at the thought of breast cancer, that I prefer not to think about it or to look for something I'd just as soon not find."

The modified radical mastectomy (removal of the breast, along with some underlying muscle and lymph nodes) is the traditional treatment for breast cancer in the U.S. But according to new evidence, this mutilating surgery may not be necessary in every case. One important five-year study showed that women whose breast lumps were small (less than 1½ inches in diameter) and whose cancers had not spread to adjacent areas did just as well with a lumpectomy (removal of the lump and a margin of surrounding tissue), plus radiation therapy.[12] The National Cancer Institute estimates that of the 119,000 women expected to have breast cancer each year, half could be candidates for the less disfiguring surgery.[13] Though more long-term research has to be done in this area, it now seems that finding a cancerous lump in its early stages may enable you to avoid the loss of a breast.

The breast self-exam should be practiced monthly. If you are still menstruating, do your exam a week after the start of your period, when there is least swelling and the breasts are easiest to examine. If you are past menopause, pick a time of the month that's easiest for you to remember (some women choose the first day of each month, or their birth dates).

There are three parts to the exam:

1. *Visual inspection.* Stand in front of the mirror with your arms at your sides. Inspect your breasts for any changes. Do you see any differences in skin color or texture? Do your nipples look red, sore or scaly? Do they pull inwardly? Next examine your breast contours in each of the following positions: 1) With your hands clasped behind your head. 2) With your hands on your hips and pressing downward. 3) While bent over slightly. Your breasts should be basically the same size and shape (although it is not uncommon for one breast to be

Breast Self Exam

There are three parts to the exam.

I. Visual inspection (in front of a mirror)

Examine your breasts for obvious changes in color and texture of skin.

Your breasts should look basically the same shape while assuming each of three positions: hands clasped behind your head; hands pressed firmly on hips; bending forward slightly.

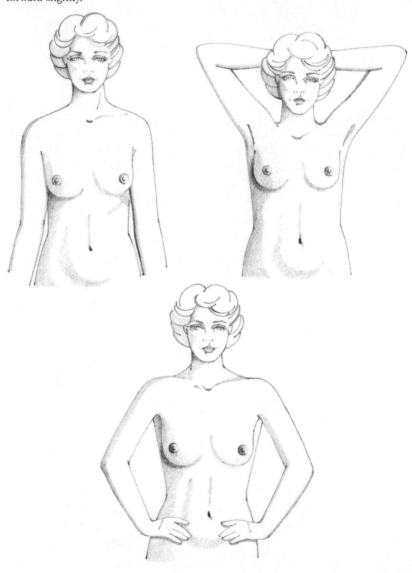

II. Lying down

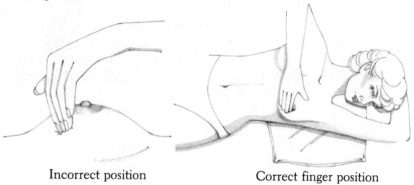

Incorrect position   Correct finger position

Correct finger position: With fingers close together, apply light and then deeper pressure. Use the pads of your fingers—not just your fingertips.

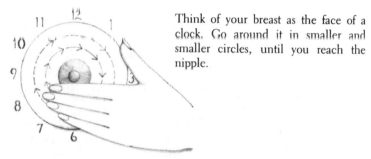

Think of your breast as the face of a clock. Go around it in smaller and smaller circles, until you reach the nipple.

When the entire breast has been covered, gently squeeze the nipple.

III. Sitting up

You may want to do this part in the shower. Do not neglect your underarm area.

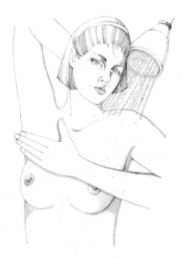

slightly larger than the other). There should be no unusual puckering, dimpling or bulges.

2. *Lie on your back.* You may want to apply lotion to your hands before doing this part. It helps your fingers to glide over your skin and to more easily feel the underlying tissue. Place a pillow or folded towel under your right shoulder and put your right hand behind your head. With your left hand examine your right breast, taking care to keep your fingers flat and pressed together. With the pads of your fingers—not your fingertips—you apply light and then deeper pressure to all areas of your breast, moving your fingers in a circular motion. Think of your breast as the face of a clock. Begin to make circles around the outermost edge of your breast, beginning at the twelve o'clock position. Then go all around until you return again to the twelve o'clock spot. Next move your fingers inward approximately one finger width toward the nipple and repeat. When the entire breast has been covered, gently squeeze your nipple to make sure that there is no discharge. Don't neglect to examine the area between your breast and armpit, including the armpit as well. Repeat these procedures in reverse for your other breast.

3. *Sitting up.* While sitting erect, place your right hand behind your head and examine your right breast exactly as described above. Repeat for the other breast. You may want to perform this part of the exam when you bathe or shower. Soapy hands make it easier to feel the texture of breast tissue.

Benign Breast Lumps

Your breasts are anything but smooth inside. They contain glands and tissues that change in shape and consistency in response to your hormone levels. Almost every woman is sure to feel a lump or grainy area in her breast at some time in her life—especially as she grows older.

Ninety percent of lumps are not cancerous.[14] Most are caused by a benign condition known as fibrocystic disease or chronic mastitis. Fibrocystic lumps are made up of enlarged fibrous tissue or of cysts that become filled with fluid. The lumps fluctuate with the menstrual cycle, becoming larger and more tender right before a woman's period and smaller right after. Larger cysts are round and firm, like the feel of an eyeball through a closed eyelid.

Women between the ages of thirty-five and fifty are most apt to have problems with this lumpy condition. It may get progressively worse until menopause. Then, when the glands shrink and the breasts become softer, the condition disappears.

Fibrocystic disease is clearly prominent in at least half of all women. Many authorities say that it is, in fact, the normal condition of the breasts—and should not be labeled as a "disease" at all.[15] Fibrocystic lumps are completely benign and do not threaten a woman's health. The major problem is that they are sometimes difficult to distinguish from cancerous lumps and may cause a woman unnecessary mental anguish.

"When the surgeon said that he wanted to remove the lump right away I almost fell off the table. 'This can't be happening to me,' I thought. I've always been healthy as a horse. We talked about which hospital I preferred, and the type of anaesthesia. Then I walked out to my car in the parking lot and cried. I had to wait two weeks until my scheduled biopsy. In that time I lost six pounds and couldn't sleep at all. The biopsy turned out negative. I am told that the lump was a fibrous swelling due to fibrocystic disease. Though I am grateful for that, I feel it's a crime to have been put through such an emotional wringer."

There is some controversy over whether women with fibrocystic disease are at higher risk for cancer. Many researchers now believe that the condition is too prevalent to be considered a risk factor.

Some women find that their fibrocystic lumps become smaller or disappear when they eliminate caffeine-containing foods and beverages from their diets (see caffeine chart on pages 83–84). Sometimes the difference is immediate, but often it takes several months for any noticeable results. Claims have also been made for supplementation with vitamins A, E and B$_6$.[16] The drug Danazol, a synthetic male hormone, makes painful breast lumps disappear, but it can also cause unpleasant masculinizing side effects and is extremely costly.[17]

Other benign breast lumps include:

• *Lipomas:* Single, painless lumps that appear most often in older women. They are soft, slow-growing, movable and are made up of fatty tissue.

• *Fibroadenomas:* Usually nontender, firm, rubbery, movable and frequently oval shaped. This type of lump is made of fibrous (fibro) and gland (adenoma) tissue. It is most commonly seen in young women between eighteen and thirty-five years old and is twice as common among blacks.

• *Fat necrosis:* A firm, round, painless mass, with redness of overlying skin, caused by a bruise or blow to the breast.

• *Intraductal papilloma:* A wartlike growth in a milk duct that usually causes a nipple discharge, and can be felt as a small nodule near the edge of the nipple.

How do you know if a lump is potentially cancerous? Your breasts are pretty much the mirror image of each other. If both of your breasts feel grainy or lumpy in the same exact area, chances are you are feeling the natural structure of your breasts. A lump or thickening is suspect if you have never felt it before, and if there's an obvious difference between the feel or contours of one breast and the other. Cancerous lumps are not usually painful, and they do not disappear after a menstrual period. Pain or tenderness in just one breast may also signal a problem. And so may nipple discharge.

What to Do When You Find a Lump

If you find a suspicious breast lump, try not to panic. Remember, 90 percent of all lumps are noncancerous. The lump may well be due to hormonal fluctuations, and disappear on its own. Your physician may tell you to watch the lump carefully for one or two menstrual cycles. Any lump that doesn't disappear by then, however, should be examined by a doctor. If you are no longer menstruating and find a lump, you should seek medical attention right away. Women past menopause are at highest risk for breast cancer.

Many women delay going to their physicians because they are afraid that they may indeed have cancer. These feelings are understandable, but postponement of medical care is actually self-defeating. When cancer is found in its early stages it is often more highly curable. You may also be able to avoid more mutilating surgery.

The physician will examine your breasts to see whether the lump "feels" cancerous. Cancerous lumps are usually harder, more irregularly shaped and less movable than benign lumps. However, it is not possible to tell with any final certainty whether the lump is cancerous unless a biopsy is done. Before recommending a biopsy, a physician may advise you to watch the lump for several cycles to see if it enlarges or disappears; or he or she may recommend one or several of the following diagnostic procedures.

• *Needle Aspiration:* This procedure may be done in the doctor's office; it helps to determine whether the lump is solid or fluid-filled. A fine needle is inserted into the lump and fluid is removed. In many cases, the cyst collapses, and that's all the treatment that is needed. The fluid may be sent to a lab

Needle Aspiration

A needle is inserted into the lump. If the lump is a fluid-filled cyst, it collapses.

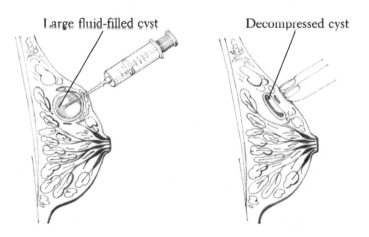

Large fluid-filled cyst   Decompressed cyst

for analysis just to reconfirm that the lump was benign. (If the cyst recurs, a repeat aspiration may have to be done, and a biopsy may be recommended.)

• *Mammography:* A mammogram is an X ray of the breast. Low levels of radiation are used to make a picture of the breast—either on X-ray film, or on paper (also called xero-mammography). This technique is so sensitive that it can show cancers that are still too small to be felt. Results are easiest to interpret in menopausal women, since their breasts are less dense than those of women in their reproductive years. If the mammogram is negative, there is a 90 percent chance that the lump is not cancerous.[18] However, a biopsy will still have to be performed for total assurance.

Most doctors would agree that a woman with a suspicious breast lump should have a mammogram. Whether or not symptom-free women should be routinely screened for breast lumps this way is another matter. Those in favor of routine mammography point to its ability to detect cancer tumors way before they can be felt manually. An earlier diagnosis means a better chance for survival. Opponents feel that the radiation—though low—is cumulative and that routine mammograms may actually cause breast cancers.[19] Another criticism is that mammography may lead to unnecessary mastectomies: some of the cancers detected by mammography are so small and slow-growing that they may never progress to a problem stage in a woman's lifetime anyway.[20]

Most major medical organizations recommend a baseline mammogram at age thirty-five to forty; however, they disagree on how often repeat mammograms should be taken thereafter. It is generally felt that women at highest risk for breast cancer, including all women over fifty, would benefit most from annual mammograms. The benefits of annual mammography for women under fifty are more questionable.

• *Ultrasonography:* High-frequency sound waves are bounced off of the breast, creating a visual image of the breast's interior. The ultrasound image helps to distinguish whether the breast lump is a solid mass or a fluid-filled cyst. Some physicians recommend an ultrasound before performing a needle aspiration.

• *Thermography:* Heat patterns from the breast are

recorded on special photographic film. Cancerous lumps are warmer than areas of normal breast tissue, and show up as a different color. The use of thermography is still experimental, and some practitioners use it as an adjunct to mammography.

• *Diaphanography:* A strong light is shone through the breast. Spots that glow red are cysts; dark spots are cancer. This method is not as accurate as mammography in discovering small cancers. It, too, may be used in conjunction with mammography.

Breast Biopsy

If, after undergoing the above diagnostic procedures, your breast lump looks the least bit suspicious, your doctor will recommend that you have a breast biopsy. This is the only surefire way to rule out a malignancy.

During the surgical biopsy the doctor makes a small incision and removes all or part of the lump for laboratory analysis. If the lump is small, it is usually removed in its entirety; if it's large, only a portion of it may be excised. It's also possible to have a needle biopsy—a small sample of tissue is obtained by a hollow needle inserted into the lump. This leaves less scarring than a surgical biopsy. But it's also less accurate, because the needle may miss the portion of the lump containing cancerous tissue. Results of a needle biopsy can only be trusted when cancer is found.

A surgical biopsy can be done under a general anaesthetic or, if the lump is not too large or deep, under a local. It's always better to go with a local if you can. There are less possible complications and fewer unpleasant side effects from the anaesthesia. One woman who had the entire lump removed under a local describes it this way: "The surgeon injected my breast with a Novocaine-like substance, and it went completely numb almost immediately. I was draped in such a way that I couldn't see the surgery. And I didn't feel any pain at all. I liked feeling in control and hearing and seeing all that was going on. I joked with the surgeon and the nurse during the entire operation. And the doctor told me right then and there that the breast tissue looked very healthy. He even held it up for me to see. (That was the only part I found a little hard to take.) I got right off the table when the procedure was over and, though a little queasy from the whole experience, was able to go out to lunch afterwards with my husband."

The biopsy incision is usually made along the curve of your breast so that it doesn't leave too noticeable a scar. Your breast may be swollen and black and blue for a time after the operation, but it will return to its natural contours after it has had time to heal. Repeated biopsies, however, may leave the breasts looking pitted. In addition, scar tissue from the operation can make it hard to examine the breasts for lumps.

Many surgeons commonly practice what is known as a one-step biopsy procedure. The biopsied breast tissue is quick frozen and examined on the spot. If cancer is diagnosed, the affected breast is removed while the woman is still under general anaesthesia. With this approach, a woman going in for a biopsy never knows for sure whether or not she'll still have her breast when she awakens.

The National Cancer Institute, as well as other agencies and experts in the field, feels that biopsy and treatment should be done in two separate stages. Their thinking is that a short delay will not make much difference in a cancer that has been growing for many years. And the additional time allows for a more thorough and accurate analysis of the biopsy tissue sample, plus more testing to assess how far the cancer has spread. If the cancer has already spread extensively, a mastectomy may be deemed unnecessary. If the cancer is in its early stages, less extreme surgery may be possible. The two-stage biopsy also gives a woman time to adjust to the fact that she has breast cancer, plus the opportunity to participate in decisions about her care. In addition, she has the chance to get a second opinion, if she so desires. (For advice on getting a second opinion, see the section at the end of this chapter.)

Some cancerous tumors are stimulated by estrogen and their growth can be controlled by medications that depress estrogen production. There is a special test—the estrogen receptor assay test—which can determine whether a tumor is estrogen-dependent or not. This test must be done on breast tissue immediately after it is removed at biopsy. Any delay can make it difficult to diagnose the cancer later. For this reason it's important that a woman find out before her biopsy whether such a test is being planned.

Bleeding Irregularities

Menstrual irregularities bring more women to the gynecologist's office than any other problem.[21] Most women in their thirties and forties begin to notice changes in their menstrual cycles. In the five to seven years before menopause, these changes become most pronounced. Periods may come closer together or further apart, or else they may come at irregular and unpredictable intervals. Bleeding may be heavier than usual or just a light stain. These changes, for the most part, are normal. They are a response by your body to declining estrogen levels and to the fact that your cycles are becoming anovulatory (without eggs). Only 10 percent of all women have regular menstrual cycles up to the age of menopause.[22]

Although premenopausal changes in your usual menstrual patterns should not be a source of undue alarm, some menstrual changes do require medical attention; notably, mid-cycle spotting or prolonged or excessive bleeding that leaves you weak or anemic. After menopause, any sort of vaginal bleeding requires prompt medical investigation, as it can be an early symptom of uterine cancer.

If you are on estrogen replacement therapy, you should be receiving regular ongoing medical monitoring. (See Chapter 6, Estrogen Therapy.) Although relatively safe in today's lower dosages, unopposed estrogen can cause an excessive buildup of the uterine lining and an increased risk of uterine cancer. Any vaginal bleeding that occurs when a woman is on estrogen should be reported immediately to her physician. Women who are on estrogen-progesterone combination therapy may have some scanty withdrawal bleeding during the drug-free period each month. This scheduled bleeding is considered normal.

Sometimes postmenopausal bleeding is caused by the thinning and drying of vaginal tissues. The fragile vaginal walls are easily injured and prone to infection. They may bleed easily, especially after intercourse. Estrogen cream or oral estrogen may be prescribed to help heal the vaginal tissue (see Chapter 6, Estrogen Therapy, for more details).

Abnormal vaginal bleeding may also be caused by the following:

Cervical or Uterine Polyps

Polyps are benign growths of excess tissue that appear on the uterine lining or cervical canal. They are usually tear-shaped and dangle from a thin stem. There may be one or several of them present. They can cause spotting between periods, heavy periods or bleeding after douching or intercourse. Cervical polyps can be felt or seen during a pelvic exam and are easily removed with forceps in the doctor's office. Uterine polyps are hidden from view, unless they extend down through the cervix. They can only be diagnosed during a D & C, at which time they may also be removed with forceps. Some polyps are flat and have no stem. Their removal is more involved and may require hospitalization.

Fibroids

One third of all women eventually have fibroids.[23] These are normally harmless growths that develop in or on the muscular wall of the uterus. Fibroids are usually detected by a physician while he or she is doing a pelvic exam. Most fibroids don't cause any symptoms and do not need to be removed. The physician just keeps an eye on them to make sure that they don't increase in size. If a fibroid does become extremely large, it may press on adjacent organs and cause such problems as stress incontinence or constipation. Though not usual, large fibroids can also cause backaches, menstrual cramping, prolonged bleeding and the passage of clots.

When fibroids cause extreme bleeding or pain they may have to be removed. A younger woman who desires more children might opt for a myomectomy—a procedure that removes the tumor but leaves the uterus in place. Physicians usually recommend that a woman over forty have a hysterectomy instead. The myomectomy is a more difficult operation than a hysterectomy and has an increased complication rate. In addition, fibroids grow back in 10 percent of all cases.[24]

Fibroids appear to be estrogen-dependent. They are most common during a woman's reproductive years, when estrogen levels are high. Their growth tends to be stimulated when a woman is on oral contraceptives or is taking estrogen replacement therapy. If you are nearing menopause and have so far managed to avoid having surgery for problem fibroids, you may want to try to bear with the condition a while longer. Most fibroids shrink after menopause.

Adenomyosis

Pieces of the uterine lining, which are usually shed each month, become embedded in the muscular wall of the uterus. There they swell each month with the menstrual cycle. The condition usually affects women between forty and fifty who have previously borne children. It can result in an enlarged and tender uterus, prolonged, heavy bleeding and menstrual pain. Adenomyosis is very difficult to diagnose without examining the uterus itself during surgery. If symptoms are very severe, a hysterectomy may be recommended. However, the condition usually improves by itself once a woman reaches menopause.

Dysfunctional Uterine Bleeding (DUB)

This is a catchall term to describe abnormal bleeding from hormonal causes. Most women with DUB don't ovulate. Failure to ovulate is very common during the last few years before menopause. When an egg fails to be released, no corpus luteum is formed, and no progesterone is produced. Progesterone normally helps the uterus to shed its lining. Thus, in an anovulatory cycle, the uterine lining may become overgrown. Bits and pieces of it may shed at various times during the cycle, and periods may be heavier than usual. If the bleeding is extremely heavy, a physician may prescribe a synthetic form of progesterone for several months. This often acts as a medical curettage. It helps the lining to shed its excess cells and may end the bleeding problem. In some cases of DUB, ovulation does occur, but the life span of the corpus luteum is abnormally short or long. Periods may be very frequent or far apart.

Sometimes an overgrowth of the uterus occurs in menopausal women who are taking estrogen. The usual course is to stop estrogen treatment, lower the dosage or add progesterone to the therapy.

Uterine Cancer

One of uterine cancer's early warning signals is mid-cycle spotting or postmenopausal bleeding. It is therefore vitally important that women seek medical care when these symptoms appear. Uterine cancer is most common among women over forty. High-risk factors include problems with fertility, a history of irregular periods, failure to ovulate and obesity. A Pap test cannot detect cancer of the uterus with a great deal of accuracy. To make a definite diagnosis, the physician will have to take a sample of the endometrial lining either via a D & C or endometrial biopsy.

Endometriosis

Material from the uterine lining somehow travels outside of the uterus and attaches itself to other surfaces. It may be found on the outside of the uterus or on other organs such as the fallopian tubes, ovaries, bladder and rectum. This misplaced endometrial tissue acts just like normal uterine lining. It swells, thickens and bleeds during the menstrual cycle. The problem is found most often in women between twenty-five and forty-five. Obvious symptoms are extremely painful menstrual cramping and pain during intercourse. Endometriosis is a common cause of infertility. It can also cause periods to become more profuse, frequent and irregular. The condition can be detected by laparoscopy (a slender telescopelike instrument is inserted through a small abdominal incision, permitting the doctor a view of the abdominal cavity). Treatment involves hormone therapy or surgery. The male hormone Danazol has been used to treat the condition with some success. However, as previously mentioned, it can have permanently masculinizing effects. Endometriosis usually ceases being a problem after menopause, when hormones no longer stimulate the uterine lining.

Cervical Cancer

Early cervical cancer is generally symptom-free, but can be easily detected by means of an annual Pap smear. As we've already mentioned, the cure rate nears 100 percent if detected at an early stage. When the disease has progressed to a more serious stage, symptoms may include staining or spotting and irregular bleeding.

Ovarian Cancer

This is a relatively rare form of cancer, yet it is the leading cause of death from gynecologic cancers. That's because there is no good way of screening women for the disease. The ovaries are hard to examine, and the initial stages of the cancer are usually symptom-free. Abdominal pain and gas may be the first symptom of the disease and later, when the tumor becomes quite large, there may be abnormal menstrual bleeding, or postmenopausal bleeding. Treatment involves removal of the ovaries, fallopian tubes and uterus.

Diagnostic Procedures

When you go to a physician because of menstrual irregularities, he or she will want to give you a thorough exam as outlined at the beginning of this chapter. You may be asked by your doctor to record your basal body temperature for a cycle or two to determine if you are ovulating. A small percentage of women experience scant bleeding at the start of pregnancy. Excessive menstrual bleeding and spotting between periods are common among IUD users. So either of these possibilities should be ruled out as causes for abnormal bleeding.

If you are under forty, but showing symptoms of menopause, your blood may be analyzed to measure the height of follicle-stimulating hormone (FSH) levels. FSH levels rise following menopause; and while such blood measurements aren't totally conclusive, they may give the physician some clue as to whether premature menopause is responsible for your menstrual abnormalities.

When there is no clear explanation for abnormal menstrual bleeding, a woman is usually advised to undergo one of the following diagnostic procedures:

Dilation and Curettage (D&C)

The cervix is opened by inserting a series of dilators—one larger than the other. A long, thin, spoon-shaped instrument called a curette is then introduced into the uterus and used to scrape the outer layer of cells on the uterine lining. If you are premenopausal, you will probably be asked to schedule your D & C during the latter part of your menstrual cycle. An examination of your uterine lining at this time permits your doctor to tell whether or not you are ovulating.

D & Cs are the second most frequent operation in the U.S., and some feel that they might be performed to excess.[25] There are some risks involved, including complications from anaesthesia and puncture of the uterus. However, when done properly, the risks are low, and the procedure can yield some very important information. D & Cs are valuable in diagnosing fibroids, uterine polyps and uterine cancer.

Some doctors prefer to do D & Cs when a woman has a general anesthesia. With the woman's muscles more completely relaxed, they feel they can do a more thorough job. Other physicians will perform a D & C in their office with a local anaesthetic. According to one physician, "The women in my practice who request a local are able to tolerate the discomfort very well. I myself prefer it because you eliminate general anaesthesia, which entails more risks than the D & C itself." Concurs one of his patients: "I found it a lot less anxiety-producing to walk into my doctor's office and have the D & C than I would have if I had to go to the hospital and be put out."

If you are going to have a D & C done with a local, your doctor may prescribe an anti-cramping drug, like Anaprox, to be taken prior to the procedure. The most uncomfortable part of the D & C will probably be the administration of the local, used to block pain in the cervix as it is being dilated. Slow, regular deep breathing during the D & C will help you to relax your pelvic muscles. The entire procedure should not last longer than ten or fifteen minutes. You may have some spotting for a few days afterward. Some women experience mild cramping as well.

Endometrial Aspiration (also known as an Aspiration Biopsy or Suction Curettage)

A thin, hollow tube called a cannula is inserted through the cervix into the uterus where it removes the uterine lining via suction. The lining can then be examined in a lab. En-

Dilatation and Curettage (D&C)

The cervix is dilated and the uterine cavity is scraped. The procedure may be done with a local or a general anesthetic. It is useful in diagnosing polyps, fibroids and uterine cancer.

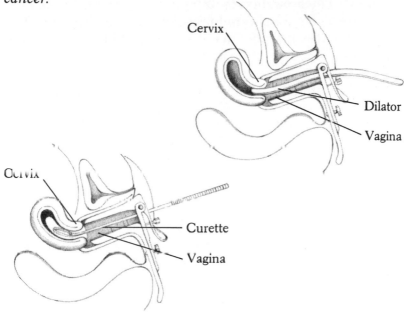

Aspiration Biopsy

The uterine lining is removed by suction.

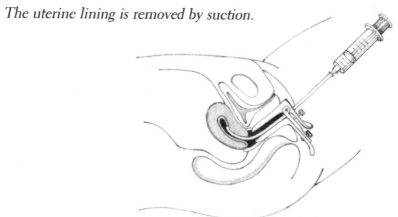

dometrial aspiration is less expensive than a D & C and there's less discomfort and risk involved. Since the cervix doesn't have to be as widely dilated, it can usually be done in the doctor's office with a local anaesthetic. Some women experience cramping during the procedure and for a few minutes afterward. The aspiration technique may be used to examine the uterine lining for abnormal thickening or to diagnose uterine cancer. It is not effective for locating fibroids or uterine polyps.

Endometrial Biopsy

An instrument is inserted through the cervix and into the uterus to obtain a small sample of endometrial lining. This is an office procedure and does not require dilation of the cervix or use of an anaesthetic. Some women experience mild cramping after it is performed. An endometrial biopsy may miss a cancerous area of the uterus, and is therefore not considered an effective diagnostic technique for uterine cancer. It may, however, be helpful in detecting hormonal imbalances, and is useful for monitoring uterine changes in women on estrogen therapy.

Colposcopy

A colposcope is a relatively new magnifying instrument that looks like a pair of binoculars mounted on a tripod. It is used to examine the cervix when Pap smears indicate the possibility of cancer. The cervix is often stained first with a solution that highlights abnormal cells. During the procedure the doctor inserts a speculum and light from the colposcope is beamed directly on the cervix. The colposcope is so powerful that it permits the physician to see cell abnormalities not evident to the naked eye. Areas that appear abnormal may be biopsied with a device that looks like a paper punch. Colposcopy is painless and can be done in a physician's office. The punch biopsy, however, may cause pain and cramping during the procedure. There may also be spotting afterward.

Conization or Cone Biopsy

This is a more extreme method of obtaining cervical tissue for biopsy. Since the advent of colposcopy, it is being used far less frequently. Conization involves the removal of a cone-

Endometrial Biopsy

A small sample of uterine tissue is taken for analysis.

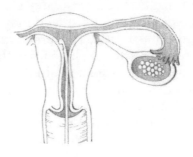

Cervical Biopsy

Punch method: *A suspicious area of tissue may be punched out.*

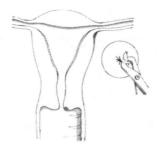

Cone method: *A cone-shaped section is removed. This is major surgery and must be performed in the hospital*

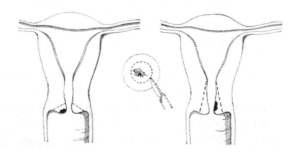

shaped section of the cervix. It is a major surgical procedure and must be done in a hospital under general anaesthesia. Heavy bleeding and infections are common postoperative complications. Conization can also make it difficult for a woman to hold a pregnancy to term, and may adversely affect mucous production. Currently, this procedure must still be used when cancerous cells are too high up in the cervical canal to be seen. If the incised section contains all of the cancerous cells, and the disease has not spread beyond the cervix, conization may be a treatment for cancer as well. Hysteretomy, however, is usually the preferred treatment for women past childbearing age, as there is always the possibility of a recurrence.

Hysterectomy

Your chances of having a hysterectomy sometime in your life are high: as it stands now, over 60 percent of all women have their wombs removed by the time they reach seventy.[26] Hysterectomy is the most frequent major operation performed in the U.S. today. Approximately 650,000 are done each year— mostly on women under forty-five years of age.[27] One expert figures that one of every four menopausal women reach menopause as a result of surgery.[28]

A hysterectomy done for the right reasons can be lifesaving. It can offer great relief from conditions that cause extreme pain or hemorrhaging. However, it has been estimated that as many as 30 to 50 percent of these operations are unnecessary.[29]

It is sometimes assumed that women don't really need their wombs once their families are complete. "If in doubt, take it out," is the dictum of many health professionals. And while they're at it, they take the ovaries, too—to prevent the possibility of future disease. In many cases a hysterectomy is performed even though other, less extreme measures might also solve the problem.

The reproductive organs do not become unnecessary once the desire for baby-making is past. And the long-range consequences of a hysterectomy are many. Some women become depressed after the operation and feel less feminine or attractive. There may be hormonal and physiologic changes that alter a woman's ability to enjoy sex. (See Chapter 9, Sexuality.) Finally, hysterectomy—with or without removal of the ovaries—can raise a premenopausal woman's chance for heart disease threefold.[30]

When the ovaries are taken along with the uterus, a premenopausal woman may be plunged into an immediate and severe menopause. Her hot flashes are likely to be intense, and her vaginal lining may become very thin and dry. She also becomes a prime candidate for osteoporosis. Removal of the ovaries in women past menopause will not have as drastic an effect—but it will still alter a woman's body chemistry. The menopausal woman's ovaries continue to produce important amounts of male hormones which are converted to estrogen elsewhere in the body.

When the uterus is removed, but the ovaries remain intact, a younger woman will most likely continue to produce estrogen and progesterone until her natural menopause. She should have all of the usual monthly menstrual changes (breast tenderness, mood swings, bloating) even though she no longer menstruates. There are exceptions to this rule. In some cases, the surgical procedure itself can interfere with the blood supply to the ovaries, and cause them to stop functioning. So even though she still has her ovaries, a woman may have menopausal symptoms.

Any major surgery involving general anaesthesia has its risks. One fourth to one half of all women undergoing a hysterectomy develop complications, with fever and hemorrhage being the most common. The mortality rate is low—600 women a year die from hysterectomies or from underlying conditions.[31]

The following conditions justify a hysterectomy:

• Cancers of the cervix, uterus, ovaries and fallopian tubes.
• Fibroids that are pressing against adjacent organs or that cause uncontrollable bleeding that cannot be helped by hormones or curettage.
• Severely diseased and infected ovaries or fallopian tubes.
• A prolapsed uterus that has descended through the vaginal opening.
• Severe endometriosis that doesn't respond to other treatments.

• Cancers or infections of adjacent organs which can't be controlled.

• Severe complications following childbirth, including postpartum hemorrhage or uterine rupture.

Hysterectomy should *not* be considered for any of the following reasons:

• As a permanent form of birth control. (A tubal ligation is a far simpler and less risky sterilization procedure.)

• To remove fibroids that cause few or no symptoms. Unless a fibroid causes a great deal of pain and bleeding, or is encroaching on other organs, it can be left in place. Some physicians base their decisions on the size of the fibroid. For example, they may suggest that a fibroid be removed when the uterus reaches the size of a twelve- or sixteen-week pregnancy. If a woman is near menopause, however, the fibroid may soon shrink in size.

• As a treatment for dysfunctional uterine bleeding that causes mild problems. Hysterectomy should only be considered if the bleeding is so severe that it is life-threatening, and only after a D & C or hormone therapy have first been tried. Often progestins can control heavy bleeding problems until menopause occurs.

• To treat a prolapsed uterus when it causes few or no symptoms.

• For prevention of possible future cancer in the absence of any disease.

Questions to Ask Your Doctor Before Surgery

The terms "partial," "total" or "complete" hysterectomy may mean different things to different doctors. A hysterectomy may involve removal of the uterus; the uterus and cervix; the uterus, cervix, ovaries and fallopian tubes; and (in rare cases of widespread cancer) removal of all the pelvic reproductive organs, plus the upper part of the vagina. When one or both ovaries and fallopian tubes are removed, the procedure is called a unilateral or bilateral salpingo-oophorectomy. Since medical terms can be confusing, ask your doctor to clearly explain which organs the hysterectomy will involve and to provide you with a diagram as well.

A hysterectomy is usually done through an abdominal incision when large tumors and ovaries are to be removed. However, the uterus can be removed vaginally in cases of severe uterine prolapse. Vaginal hysterectomies have lower complication rates, and a woman usually recovers from them more quickly. Not all doctors are skilled in this method, however; in improper hands a vaginal hysterectomy may increase a woman's risk of urinary tract injury. It may also leave her vagina shortened, and cause discomfort during intercourse.[32]

When faced with this—or any other kind of surgery—you might want to ask your doctor the following questions:

1. Why do I need this surgery?
2. What are the risks or possible complications from the operation? What are the benefits?
3. Can I live with this condition, or will it worsen over time?
4. How long can I safely go without having the operation?
5. What will happen if I decide against the surgery?
6. Are there any alternative treatments?
7. What risks do these treatments entail?
8. What exactly will be done to me during the operation?
9. What type of anaesthesia will be used? What are the possible risks with this type of anaesthesia?
10. How long a hospital stay can I expect?
11. Will there be much postoperative discomfort?
12. How long until I can resume normal activities?

Getting a Second Opinion

No matter how much you like and respect your doctor, you should always seek a second or even third opinion regarding the need for major treatments or surgery. There are wide disagreements over medical approaches among even the best physicians.

You may feel hesitant about getting another opinion for fear that you may offend your physician. But any doctor worth his salt will react with understanding. Even if feelings are ruffled, you must consider where your priorities lie. This is your body and your future health may be at stake. You can be sure that many doctors themselves seek several opinions before they agree to undergo serious surgery. One doctor from a small city says that when he was seriously ill he flew to a large metropolitan area to seek the opinions of several prominent medical experts. If you can't muster enough courage to tell your physician, go and get your second opinion anyway. While it's always best to be honest, the main thing is that you seek the medical care that you need.

Finding another doctor can be a tricky task. As in any other profession, some doctors are more competent than others. How do you judge? You might get a referral from a friend who has beliefs about health care that are similar to yours. Or you might want to try to locate a physician on staff at a university teaching hospital. Your county medical society can provide you with the names of several physicians in a particular specialty, and they may also be able to provide information about their educational background and professional affiliations. Information on physicians' credentials can also be obtained in the following directories, available in most public libraries: *The American College of Surgeons Yearbook*, *The Directory of Medical Specialties* and *The American Medical Directory of the American Medical Association*. However, it's up to you to screen these doctors either over the phone or during an initial consultation. It may cost you the price of several office visits before you settle on a physician that you trust, but when the price is your health, it may be worth it in the long run.

Here are some basic guidelines to keep in mind when shopping around for a second opinion:

• Don't ask the first doctor for a referral. Try to find a physician who is located in a different hospital, and who has no affiliation with your doctor. This will help to guarantee a more impartial assessment of your case. If you live in a very small town, consider going to another city.

• Surgeons will naturally recommend surgery—that's what they are trained to do. For a different perspective on treatment options, consider seeing a doctor from another specialty, such as an internist.

• Be up front with the new physician: tell him or her that you have a health problem and are seeking a second opinion. Since this physician will not be involved in your treatment, he or she is more likely to give you an unbiased diagnosis. It is probably best if you don't name your original physician, or tell what the preliminary diagnosis was until the end of your office visit. That way the physician can't be swayed by professional loyalties.

• Go to the library and read up, as much as possible, about your particular condition. This will help you to intelligently discuss your options with the doctor, and evaluate more fully the advice he or she gives.

• Often when you have a physical problem, you are too rattled to wholly absorb what a doctor is saying to you. It's a good idea to bring a notebook with you and take notes on what the doctor says. You can refer to your notes later when you are in a calmer state.

• If possible, have a support person—either a friend or relative—accompany you to the consultation visit. He or she will be in a better frame of mind to ask questions, and to go over with you what was actually said in the office.

• The second opinion you receive may differ from the first. In such a case you may want to go on to get a third opinion as well.

Getting a second opinion takes a lot of effort, especially when you are already in a health crisis. It would be so much nicer if you could just sit back and let the doctor take over all the decision-making for you. Unfortunately, the easy way out is not always best. It's up to you to gather as much information as you can about all possible treatment options. Read. Ask questions. Demand clear explanations from health care providers. It pays to be a good medical consumer. As the old axiom goes: If you've got your health, you've got everything.

Conclusion

*I*f you were to choose the best time and place in history to be a middle-aged woman, the answer might well be here and now. In no other time have women lived so long, enjoyed such health and vigor, or had so many personal and career options. A woman in her forties and fifties is no longer considered "old." Attractive and confident, she may enroll for that long-postponed college education, spiff up her resume and change careers, or become an encouraging mentor for younger women in her field.

We are coming to see menopause in a new light as well. Our grandmothers may have felt as if they were obsolete when childbearing drew to an end. Today, women define themselves in much broader terms. The loss of fertility means freedom from contraceptive hassles and time for personal growth. Menopause is not the end of the line. It is just another of the many physical changes a woman goes through in her lifetime.

Myths about menopause die hard, but they are being slowly

dispelled. Scientific studies are showing that women are not unduly neurotic or depressed at menopause, and that most continue to enjoy satisfying sex well into old age. Most pass through menopause with minor discomforts and need no special medical care.

More and more lay literature is coming out on menopausal issues, and this is helping women to understand the physical changes they are going through. With healthier attitudes about sexuality, women are sharing with each other what it's really like to go through the "changes." Menopause workshops and support groups are springing up in every city. This increased knowledge brings reassurance.

Diseases and infirmities increase as we grow older. But for most, the menopausal years are a time of continued health and vitality. We know a lot more about the benefits of nutrition and exercise than did women of previous generations. If we incorporate this knowledge into our daily routines, we can help to make our middle years some of the best in our lives.

Helpful Agencies

Menopause

Many local agencies provide menopause information and group support. To find out if there are menopause workshops or support groups in your area, contact your local YMCA, YWCA, American Red Cross, family or community service agencies, women's organizations, department of health or Planned Parenthood. If you cannot locate an existing support group you may wish to form one of your own. Guidelines for doing so appear in Chapter 5, Getting "Up" and Out.

Center for Climacteric Studies
University of Florida
901 N.W. 8th Avenue
Suite B 1
Gainesville, FL 32601
Phone: (904) 392-3184

This organization is involved in research and the dissemination of information on all phases of menopause. They publish a quarterly journal, *Midlife Wellness*, that includes authoritative articles on all aspects of menopause, plus medical abstracts and book reviews. The articles are on the technical side, but are suitable for the lay reader who wants an in-depth view of the subject.

Career Guidance

Catalyst
14 East 60th Street
New York, NY 10022
Phone: (212) 759-9700

If you're thinking about returning to work or school and need some guidance, you might begin by contacting Catalyst. This nonprofit New York–based agency acts as a national referral service and can direct you to career counseling and continuing education programs in your area. They also publish helpful books and pamphlets.

Sleep Disorders

The Association of Sleep Disorders Centers
P.O. Box 2604
Del Mar, CA 92014
Phone: (619) 455-8087

This organization can direct you to sleep disorders clinics nearest you. They may be able to help you with a chronic sleep problem.

Stress

Stress reduction seminars are offered at adult education programs in high schools and universities and through many nonprofit agencies (such as the American Red Cross, family services, YMCAs and YWCAs). There is also a tape-recorded relaxation lesson, including soft-spoken instructions and soothing background music, entitled "Letting Go of Stress." The tape is distributed by the following two companies:

Source
P.O. Box W
Sanford, CA 94305
Phone: (415) 328-7171

Halpern Sounds
1775 Old County Road, No. 9
Belmont, CA 94002
Phone: (415) 592-4900

Cancer

Breast Cancer Advisory Center
Rose Kushner, Director
Box 422
Kensington, MD 20795
Phone: (301) 949-2530

Provides referrals and information on cancer, with breast cancer being its main focus.

Cancer Information Service, National Cancer Hotline
1-800-4-CANCER
In Hawaii call: (808) 524-1234
In Alaska call: 1-800-638-6070
In Washington, D.C., call: (202) 636-5700

A toll-free phone service for anyone who needs advice or information about cancer.

Reach to Recovery Program

Sponsored by the American Cancer Society. Women who've had mastectomies counsel other women after breast cancer surgery. Contact your local chapter of the American Cancer Society.

YWCA Encore

A YWCA-sponsored group offering support and exercises for women who have had mastectomies. Contact your local YWCA for the Encore group nearest you.

RENU
Phone: (216) 444-2900

A phone information service for women considering breast reconstruction surgery. Call to leave your name and number—then someone calls you back, often from your own area.

Eye Care

The American Academy of Opthalmology
1833 Fillmore Street
P.O. Box 17424
San Francisco, CA 94120
Phone: (415) 921-4700

Informative pamphlets on cataracts, glaucoma and other diseases of the eyes.

Plastic Surgery

American Academy of Facial Plastic and Reconstructive
    Surgery
70 West Hubbard Street
Suite 202
Chicago, IL 60610
Phone: (312) 644-2623

Distributes free patient education brochures on various types of cosmetic surgery.

Nutrition and Exercise

American Heart Association
7320 Greenville Avenue
Dallas, TX 75231
Phone: (214) 750-5300

National Dairy Council
6300 North River Road
Rosemont, IL 60018
Phone: (312) 696-1020

The American Heart Association has literature on nutrition and exercise. The National Dairy Council puts out a wide range of educational materials on nutrition, weight control and osteoporosis. You can probably get literature more quickly by visiting or calling local chapters of these organizations.

Sexuality

American Association of Sex Educators, Counselors and
   Therapists (AASECT)
11 Dupont Circle N.W., Suite 220
Washington, D.C. 20036
Phone: (202) 462-1171

This agency publishes a National Register of Certified Sex Educators and Sex Therapists and will help you find a reputable sex therapist in your area.

Women's Health Issues

Planned Parenthood Federation of America
810 Seventh Avenue
New York, NY 10019
Phone: (212) 541-7800

Literature, pamphlets, workshops, film strips on a large variety of women's topics, including menopause. Contact your local branch to see what services are available in your area.

The National Women's Health Network
224 Seventh Street, S.E.
Washington, D.C. 20003
Phone: (202) 223-6886

A national consumer organization devoted to women and health. Members get monthly newsletters on latest developments in women's health care and can avail themselves of a national resource file on various health topics.

General Health Information

Consumer Information Centers
P.O. Box 100
Pueblo, CO 81002

Send for their *Consumer Information Catalog,* a list of useful booklets from more than thirty agencies of the federal government. They will send you as many as twenty-five titles for free, plus other publications that are reasonably priced. Among topics: careers and education, nutrition, health, exercise, mental health.

Suggested Reading

Menopause—Professional Books

Buchsbaum, Herbert J., ed. *The Menopause.* New York: Springer-Verlag, 1983.

Eskin, Bernard A., ed. *The Menopause: Comprehensive Management.* Masson Publishers, 1980.

Greene, John G. *The Social and Psychological Origins of the Climacteric Syndrome.* Brookfield, Vt.: Gower Publishing Co., 1984.

Haspels, A. A. and Musaph, H., eds. *Psychosomatics in Perimenopause.* Baltimore: University Park Press, 1979.

Utian, Wulf H. *Menopause in Modern Perspective.* New York: Appleton-Century-Crofts, 1980.

Voda, Ann M., Dinnerstein, Myra, and O'Donnell, Sheryl R., eds. *Changing Perspectives on Menopause.* Austin: University of Texas Press, 1982.

Career Counseling

Abarbanel, Karin and Siegel, Gonnie McClung. *Woman's Work Book.* New York: Praeger Publishers, 1975.

Bolles, Richard Nelson. *What Color Is Your Parachute?* Berkeley, Ca.: Ten Speed Press, 1983.

Bolles, Richard Nelson. *The Three Boxes of Life and How to Get Out of Them.* Berkeley, Ca.: Ten Speed Press, 1984.

Catalyst. *Marketing Yourself.* New York: G. P. Putnam's Sons, 1980.

Sumners, Jean. *What Every Woman Needs to Know to Find a Job in Today's Tough Market.* New York: Fawcett-Columbine, 1980.

Stress

Benson, Herbert. *The Relaxation Response.* New York: William Morrow & Co., 1975.

Blue Cross/Blue Shield of Maryland. *Stress.* 1974. A free 96-page booklet which can be obtained by writing to: Public Relations Dept., Blue Cross/Blue Shield of Maryland, 700 East Joppa Road, Baltimore, Maryland, 21204.
Bright, D. *Creative Relaxation: Turning Your Stress Into Positive Energy.* New York: Harcourt Brace Jovanovich, 1979.
McQuade, Walter and Aikman, Ann. *Stress.* New York: E. P. Dutton & Co., 1974.

Insomnia
Maxmen, Jerold S. *A Good Night's Sleep.* New York: W. W. Norton & Co., 1981.
Phillips, Elliott Richard. *Get a Good Night's Sleep.* Englewood Cliffs, N.J.: Prentice-Hall, Inc., 1983.
Regestein, Quentin R., with Rechs, James R. *Sound Sleep.* New York: Simon & Schuster, 1980.

Mid-Life Crisis
Donohugh, Donald L. *The Middle Years: A Physician's Guide to Your Body, Emotions and Life Challenges.* New York: Berkley Publishers, 1983.
Fuchs, Estelle. *Life, Love and Sex For Women in the Middle Years.* New York: Anchor Books, 1978.
London, Mel. *Second Spring.* Emmaus, Pa.: Rodale Press, 1982.
Sheehy, Gail. *Passages.* New York: Bantam Books, 1974.
Sheehy, Gail. *Pathfinders.* New York: William Morrow & Co., 1981.

Nutrition
Brody, Jane. *Jane Brody's Nutrition Book.* New York: W. W. Norton & Co., 1981.
Eshelman, Ruthe and Winston, Mary. *The American Heart Association Cookbook,* Fourth Revised Edition. New York: Ballantine Books, 1985.
Natow, Annette, and Heslin, Jo Ann. *Nutrition for the Prime of Your Life.* New York: McGraw-Hill, 1983.

Exercise
Devries, Herbert A., with Hales, Dianne. *Fitness After Fifty.* New York: Charles Scribner's Sons, 1982.

Kuntzleman, Charles. *The Exerciser's Handbook*. New York: David McKay, Co., Inc., 1978.

Osteoporosis
Notelovitz, Morris, and Ware, Marsha. *Stand Tall! The Informed Woman's Guide to Preventing Osteoporosis*. Gainesville, Fl.: Triad Publishing Co., 1982.

Hysterectomy
Morgan, Susanne. *Coping With a Hysterectomy*. New York: The Dial Press, 1982.

General Health
American Medical Association. *The American Medical Association Guide to Health and Well-Being After 50*. New York: Random House, 1984.
Boston Women's Health Collective. *The New Our Bodies Ourselves*. New York: Simon & Schuster, 1984.
Brody, Jane. *The New York Times Guide to Personal Health*. New York: Times Books, 1982.
Cooper, Patricia J., ed. *Better Homes and Gardens Woman's Health and Medical Guide*. Des Moines, Iowa: Meredith Corp., 1981.
Lettvin, Maggie. *Maggie's Woman's Book*. Boston: Houghton Mifflin Co., 1980.
Madaras, Lynda and Patterson, Jane. *Womancare*. New York: Avon Books, 1981.
Porcino, Jane. *Growing Older, Getting Better*. Reading, Ma.: Addison-Wesley, 1983.
Seaman, Barbara and Seaman, Gideon. *Women and the Crisis in Sex Hormones*. New York: Bantam Books, 1977.
Shephard, Bruce D., and Shephard, Carroll A. *The Complete Guide to Women's Health*. Tampa, Florida: Mariner Publishing Co., Inc., 1982.
Weideger, Paula. *Menstruation and Menopause*. New York: Delta Books, 1977.

Sexuality
Barbach, Lonnie Garfield. *For Yourself: The Fulfillment of Female Sexuality*. New York: Doubleday/Anchor Books, 1976.

Barbach, Lonnie, and Levine, Linda. *Shared Intimacies: Women's Sexual Experiences.* New York: Bantam Books, 1980.

Hite, Shere. *The Hite Report.* New York: Macmillan Publishing Co., 1976.

Kaplan, Helen S. *The Illustrated Manual of Sex Therapy.* New York: G. P. Putnam's Sons, 1983.

————. *The New Sex Therapy.* New York: Quadrangle/New York Times Book Co., 1973.

Kitzinger, Sheila. *Woman's Experience of Sex.* New York: G. P. Putnam's Sons, 1983.

Skin and Hair Care

Dvorine, William. *A Dermatologist's Guide to Home Skin Treatment.* New York: Charles Scribner's Sons, 1983.

Feinberg, Herbert S. *All About Hair.* New York: Simon & Schuster, 1979.

Gignac, Louis, and Warsaw, Jacqueline. *Everything You Need to Know to Have Great Looking Hair.* New York: The Viking Press, 1981.

Klein, Arnold W., Sternbert, James H., and Bernstein, Paul. *The Skin Book.* New York: Macmillan Pub. Co., 1980.

Schoen, Linda Allen, ed. *The AMA Book of Skin and Hair Care.* New York: J. B. Lippincott Co., 1976.

Unnecessary Surgery

Keyser, Herbert H. *Women Under the Knife.* Philadelphia: George F. Stickley Co., 1984.

Notes

Chapter 1
What Is Menopause? and Other Good Questions

1. Bonnie Pedersen and Elaine Pendleton, "Menopause: A Welcome or Dreaded Stage of Development," *Journal of Nurse Midwifery*, vol. 23 (Fall 1978), pp. 45–51.

2. *The World Almanac and Book of Facts 1984*, cites data from National Center for Health Statistics, U.S. Dept. of Health and Human Services (New York: Newspaper Enterprise Association, Inc., 1984), p. 910.

3. James L. Breen, "What Was, What Is and What May Be" (President Address at the 31st Annual Clinical Meeting of the American College of Obstetricians and Gynecologists, Atlanta, Ga., May 11, 1983).

4. Clare D. Edman, "The Climacteric," *The Menopause*, ed. Herbert J. Buchsbaum (New York: Springer-Verlag, 1983), pp. 23–33.

5. A. A. Haspels and P. A. Van Keep, "Endocrinology and Management of the Peri-Menopause," *Psychosomatics in Peri-Menopause*, ed. A. A. Haspels and H. Musaph (Baltimore: University Park Press, 1979), pp. 57–71.

6. Michael R. Soules and William J. Bremner, "The Menopause and Climacteric: Endocrinologic Basis and Associated Symptomology," *Journal of the American Geriatrics Society*, vol. 30, no. 9 (Sept. 1982), pp. 547–561.

7. Wulf H. Utian, *Menopause in Modern Perspective* (New York: Appleton-Century-Crofts, 1980).

8. Delores Hemphill and Yvonne Kimber, "A Positive Look at Menopause," *Teacher Training Manual,* Planned Parenthood of Central Missouri, 1982.

9. Pedersen and Pendleton, pp. 45–51.

10. Haspels and Van Keep, "Management of the Peri-Menopause."

11. Sonja McKinlay, Margot Jeffreys and Barbara Thompson, "An Investigation of the Age at Menopause," *Journal of Biological Science,* vol. 4 (1972), pp. 161–173.

12. Hemphill and Kimber, "Look at Menopause."

13. Linda Pearson, "Climacteric," *American Journal of Nursing,* vol. 82, no. 7 (July 1982), pp. 1098–1102.

14. F. S. Anderson, I. Transbol and C. Christiansen, "Is Cigarette Smoking a Promoter of the Menopause?" *Acta Med. Scand.,* vol. 212, no. 3 (1982), pp. 137–139.

15. W. Willet, et al., "Cigarette Smoking, Relative Weight and Menopause," *American Journal of Epidemiology,* vol. 117, no. 6 (1983), pp. 651–656.

16. Laura Ryan Caldwell, "Questions and Answers About the Menopause," *American Journal of Nursing,* vol. 82, no. 7 (July 1982), p. 1100.

17. Pedersen and Pendleton, pp. 45–51.

18. Stanley G. Korenman, "Menopausal Endocrinology and Management," *Archives of Internal Medicine,* vol. 142 (June 1982), pp. 1131–1136.

19. Wulf H. Utian, "Current Status of Menopause and Postmenopausal Estrogen Therapy," *Obstetrical and Gynecological Survey,* vol. 32, no. 4 (1977).

20. Susan A. LaRocca and Denise Polit, "Women's Knowledge About the Menopause," *Nursing Research,* vol. 29, no. 1 (February 1980), pp. 10–13.

21. Anthony H. Labrum, "Depression and Feminine Endocrine Pathology." (Unpublished paper, University of Rochester School of Medicine and Dentistry, Department of Obstetrics-Gynecology and Psychiatry, 1984).

22. Natalie Shainess, "Menopause: Midlife Crisis or Milestone Marker?" *Journal of the American Medical Women's Association,* vol. 37, no. 4 (April 1982), pp. 87–90.

23. Jean Coope, "Problems Around the Menopause," *The Practitioner,* vol. 227, no. 1379 (May 1983), pp. 793–803.

24. Caldwell, p. 1100.

25. Edman, pp. 23–33.

26. Bernice L. Neugarten and Ruth J. Kraines, "'Menopausal Symptoms' in Women of Various Ages," *Psychosomatic Medicine,* vol. 27, no. 3 (1965), pp. 266–273.

27. Mary Clare Lennon, "The Psychological Consequences of Menopause: The Importance of Timing of a Life Stage Event," *Journal of Health and Social Behavior,* vol. 23, no. 4 (Dec. 1982), pp. 353–366.

28. James. L. Breen, "Sex After 50," The American College of Obstetricians and Gynecologists, news release (Sept. 26, 1983).

29. Bernice L. Neugarten et al., "Women's Attitudes Toward the Menopause," *Vita Humana*, vol. 6 (1963), pp. 140–151.

30. Barbara Seaman and Gideon Seaman, *Women and the Crisis in Sex Hormones* (New York: Bantam Books, 1977), p.360.

31. Kathryn E. McGoldrick, "Myths, Menopause and Middle Age," *Journal of the American Medical Woman's Association*, editorial, vol. 37, no. 4 (April, 1982), p. 86.

Chapter 2
The Female Hormones

1. Michael R. Soules and William J. Bremner, "The Menopause and Climacteric: Endocrinologic Basis and Associated Symptomology," *Journal of the American Geriatrics Society*, vol. 30, no. 9 (Sept. 1982), pp. 547–561.

2. Paula Weideger, *Menstruation and Menopause* (New York: Alfred A. Knopf, 1976).

3. Clare D. Edman, "The Climacteric," *The Menopause*, ed. Herbert J. Buchsbaum (New York: Springer Verlag, 1983), pp. 23–33.

4. Weideger, *Menstruation and Menopause*.

5. Soules and Bremner, pp. 547–561.

6. Inge Dyrenfurth, "Endocrine Functions in the Woman's Second Half of Life," *Changing Perspectives on Menopause*, ed. A. Voda, M. Dinnerstein, and S. R. O'Donnell (Austin: University of Texas Press, 1982), pp. 307–334.

7. Esther C. Jones, "The Post-Fertile Life of Non-Human Primates and Other Mammals," *Psychosomatics in Peri-Menopause*, ed. A. A. Haspels and H. Musaph (Baltimore: University Park Press, 1979), pp. 13–39.

8. Soules and Bremner, pp. 547–561.

9. Edman, pp. 23–33.

10. Wulf H. Utian, *Menopause in Modern Perspective* (New York: Appleton-Century-Crofts, 1980).

11. David Archer, "Biomedical Findings and Medical Management of the Menopause," *Changing Perspectives on Menopause*, ed. A. Voda, M. Dinnerstein, and S. R. O'Donnell (Austin: University of Texas Press, 1982), pp. 39–48.

12. Soules, pp. 547–561.

13. Archer, pp. 39–48.

14. Edman, pp. 23–33.

15. Stanley G. Korenman, "Menopausal Endocrinology and Management," *Archives of Internal Medicine*, vol. 142 (June 1982), pp. 1131–1136.

16. Gary De Vane, "Hormonal Changes During the Climacteric," *Menopause Update*, vol. 1, no. 2 (1983), pp. 2–6.

17. Marcha P. Flint, "Transcultural Influences in Peri-Menopausal Research," *Psychosomatics in Peri-Menopause*, ed. A. A. Haspels, and H. Musaph (Baltimore: University Park Press, 1979), pp. 41–55.

18. Bonnie Pedersen and Elaine Pendleton, "Menopause: A Welcome or Dreaded Stage of Development," *Journal of Nurse Midwifery*, vol. 23 (Fall 1978), pp. 45–51.

19. Flint, pp. 41–55.

20. Dyrenfurth, pp. 307–334.

Chapter 3
Hot Flashes

1. American College of Obstetricians and Gynecologists, *Technical Bulletin*, no. 70 (June 1983).

2. C. J. Dewhurst, "Frequency and Severity of Menopausal Symptoms," *The Management of the Menopause and Post-Menopausal Years*, ed. Stuart Campbell (Baltimore: University Park Press, 1976), pp. 25–27.

3. Ann M. Voda, "Hot Flushes/Flashes . . . A Descriptive Analysis," *Menopause Update*, vol. 1, no. 2 (1983), pp. 17–20.

4. John S. Rhinehart and Isaac Schiff, "Hormone Imbalance: Hormone Treatment?" *Menopause Update*, vol. 1, no. 2 (1983), pp. 13–16.

5. Wulf H. Utian, "Current Status of Menopause and Postmenopausal Estrogen Therapy," *Obstetrical and Gynecological Survey*, vol. 32, no. 4 (1977), pp. 193–204.

6. Ann M. Voda, "Menopausal Hot Flash," *Changing Perspectives on Menopause*, ed. A. M. Voda, M. Dinnerstein, and S. R. O'Donnell (Austin: University of Texas Press, 1982), pp. 136–159.

7. Voda, "Hot Flushes/Flashes," pp. 17–20.

8. Leonide Martin, *Health Care of Women* (Philadelphia: J. B. Lippincott Co., 1978).

9. George W. Molnar, "Body Temperatures During Menopausal Hot Flashes," *Journal of Applied Physiology*, vol. 38, no. 3 (Mar. 1975), pp. 499–503.

10. Edward M. Davis and Dona Z. Meilach, *A Doctor Discusses Menopause and Estrogens* (Chicago: Budlong Press Co., 1981).

11. Martin, *Health Care*.

12. Molnar, pp. 499–503.

13. Voda, "Hot Flushes/Flashes," p. 17–20.

14. Rhinehart and Schiff, pp. 13–16.

15. William G. Bates, "On the Nature of the Hot Flash," *Clinical Obstetrics and Gynecology*, vol. 24, no. 1 (Mar. 1981), pp. 231–241.

16. E. Cope, "Physical Changes Associated with the Post-Menopausal Years," *The Management of the Menopause and Post-Menopausal Years*, ed. Stuart Campbell (Baltimore: University Park Press, 1976), pp. 29–42.

17. Yohanan Erlik, David R. Meldrum, and Howard L. Judd, "Estrogen Levels in Postmenopausal Women with Hot Flashes," *Obstetrics and Gynecology*, vol. 59, no. 4 (Apr. 1982), pp. 403–407.

18. Rhinehart and Schiff, pp. 13–16.

19. Isaac Schiff, "The Effects of Progestins on Vasomotor Flushes," *The Journal of Reproductive Medicine*, vol. 27, no. 8 (Aug. 1982), pp. 498–502.

20. Michael R. Soules and William J. Bremner, "The Menopause and Climacteric: Endocrinologic Basis and Associated Symptomology," *Journal of the American Geriatrics Society*, vol. 30, no. 9 (Sept. 1982), pp. 547–561.

21. Jonathan K. Wilkin, "Flushing Reactions: Consequences and Mechanisms, *Annals of Internal Medicine*, vol. 95, no. 4 (1981), pp. 468–476.

22. R. F. Casper, S. S. C. Yen and M. M. Wilkes, "Menopausal Flushes: A Neuroendocrine Link with Pulsatile Luteinizing Hormone Secretion," *Science*, vol. 205 (Aug. 24, 1979), pp. 823–825.

23. Bates, pp. 231–241.

24. Wilkin, pp. 468–476.

25. Voda, pp. 136–159.

26. Louisa Rose, ed., *The Menopause Book* (New York: Hawthorn Books Inc., 1977).

27. Pat Kaufert and John Syrotuik, "Symptom Reporting at the Menopause," *Social Science Medicine*, vol. 15E (1981), pp. 173–184.

28. Erlik, Meldrum and Judd, pp. 403–407.

29. Council on Scientific Affairs, "Council Report: Estrogen Replacement in the Menopause," *Journal of the American Medical Association*, vol. 249, no. 3 (Jan. 21, 1983), pp. 359–361.

30. Erlik, Meldrum and Judd, pp. 403–407.

31. Rhinehart and Schiff, pp. 13–16.

32. Schiff, pp. 498–502.

33. Felicia Stewart et al., *My Body My Health* (New York: John Wiley and Sons, 1979).

34. Wulf H. Utian, *Menopause in Modern Perspective* (New York: Appleton-Century-Crofts, 1980).

35. W. E. Court, "Ginseng—A Chinese Folk Medicine of Current Interest," *The Pharmaceutical Journal* (Mar. 1, 1975), pp. 180–181.

36. Dolores Hemphill and Yvonne Kimber, "A Positive Look at Menopause," *Teacher Training Manual* (Planned Parenthood of Central Missouri, 1982).

37. Maria Cristina Lopez et al., *Menopause: A Self-Care Manual* (Santa Fe, N. Mex.: Santa Fe Health Education Project, 1980).

38. Planned Parenthood of Rochester and Monroe County, "Menopause," brochure distributed 1984.

39. Barbara Seaman and Gideon Seaman, *Women and the Crisis in Sex Hormones* (New York: Bantam Books, 1977).

40. Maggie Lettvin, *Maggie's Woman's Book* (Boston: Houghton, Mifflin Co., 1980).

41. Seaman and Seaman, *Sex Hormones*.

42. Marsha Ware, "Does Vitamin E. Help Hot Flashes?," *Menopause Update*, vol. 1, no. 1 (Fall 1982), p. 33.

43. Hemphill and Kimber, "Look at Menopause."

44. Ware, p. 33.

45. Lopez, et al., *Self Care* Manual.

Chapter 4
Middle-Age Blues

1. Ellen Goodman, "Gary Makes Her Feel Young Again" (The Boston Globe Newspaper Company/Washington Post Writers Group, March 30, 1984).

2. Jean Coope, "Problems Around the Menopause," *The Practitioner*, vol. 222, no. 1379 (May 1983), pp. 793–803.

3. G. T. Bungay, M. P. Vessey and C. K. McPherson, "Study of Symptoms in Middle Life With Special Reference to the Menopause," *British Medical Journal*, vol. 281, no. 6233 (July 19, 1980), pp. 181–183.

4. Jean Coope, "Symptoms in Middle Life and the Menopause," letter, *British Medical Journal*, vol. 281, no. 6243 (Sept. 20, 1980), p. 811.

5. Anthony H. Labrum, "Depression and Feminine Endocrine Pathology" (Unpublished paper, University of Rochester School of Medicine and Dentistry, Department of Obstetrics-Gynecology and Psychology, 1984).

6. Paul J. Fink, "Psychiatric Myths of the Menopause," *The Menopause: Comprehensive Management*, ed. Bernard A. Eskin (Masson Pub., USA, 1980), pp. 111–128.

7. Planned Parenthood of Rochester and Monroe County, Inc., *My Menopause: Program Guide* (Rochester, N.Y.: Education Department Publications).

8. Marcha P. Flint, "Sociocultural Aspects of the Menopause," *Menopause Update*, vol. 1, no. 1 (Fall 1982), pp. 22–24.

9. Ibid.

10. Karen J. Armitage, Lawrence J. Schneiderman and Robert A. Bass, "Response of Physicians to Medical Complaints in Men and Women," *Journal of the American Medical Association*, vol. 241, no. 20 (May 18, 1979), pp. 2186–87.

11. Marcha P. Flint, "The Menopause: Reward or Punishment?," *Psychosomatics*, vol. 16 (Oct./Nov./Dec. 1975), pp. 161–163.

12. Flint, "Sociocultural Aspects," pp. 22–24.

13. Marcha P. Flint, "Transcultural Influences in Peri-Menopause," *Psychosomatics in Peri-Menopause*, ed. A. A. Haspels and H. Musaph (Baltimore: University Park Press, 1979), pp. 41–55.

14. Sherry Jill Tucker, "The Menopause: How Much Soma and How Much Psyche?" *JOGN Nursing*, Sept./Oct. 1977, pp. 40–48.

15. Diane Alington-MacKinnon and Lillian E. Troll, "The Adaptive Function of the Menopause: A Devil's Advocate Position," *Journal of the American Geriatrics Society*, vol. 29, no. 8 (Aug. 1981), pp. 349–353.

16. Gloria Steinem, "Fifty Is What 40 Used to Be—and Other Thoughts on Growing Up," *Ms.*, vol. 12, no. 12 (June 1984), pp. 108–110.

17. Gail Sheehy, *Pathfinders* (New York: William Morrow and Company, Inc., 1981).

Chapter 5
Getting "Up" and Out

1. Walter McQuade and Ann Aikman, *Stress* (New York: E. P. Dutton & Co., Inc., 1974).

2. Thomas H. Holmes and Richard H. Rahe, "The Social Readjustment Rating Scale," *Journal of Psychosomatic Research*, vol. 2, no. 2 (Aug. 1967), pp. 213–218.

3. Dallas Stevenson and Dennis J. Delprato, "Multiple Component Self-Control Program for Menopausal Hot Flashes," *Journal of Behavior Therapy and Experimental Psychiatry*, vol. 14, no. 2 (June, 1983), pp. 137–140.

4. Elliott Richard Phillips, *Get a Good Night's Sleep* (Englewood Cliffs, N.J.: Prentice-Hall, Inc., 1983).

5. Jerold S. Maxmen, *A Good Night's Sleep* (New York: W. W. Norton & Co., 1981).

6. Ibid.

7. Ibid.

8. Ibid.

9. Philips, *Get a Good Night's Sleep.*

10. Maxmen, *Good Night's Sleep.*

11. Louise Corbett, "Getting Our Bodies Back: Menopause Self-Help Groups" (Information sheet from The Menopause Collective, Cambridge, Mass., 1981).

12. Paul J. Fink, "Psychiatric Myths of the Menopause," *The Menopause: Comprehensive Management*, ed. Bernard A. Eskin (Masson Pub., USA, 1980), pp. 111–128

13. Ilene S. Levenson, "Research Briefs: Impact of Work on Women at Midlife," *Midlife Wellness*, vol. 1, no. 3 (1983), p. 46.

14. Liesbeth Severne, "Psychosocial Aspects of the Menopause," *Changing Perspectives on Menopause*, ed. A. Voda, M. Dinnerstein, and S. R. O'Donnell (Austin: University of Texas Press, 1982), pp. 239–247.

Chapter 6
Estrogen Therapy: Yes or No?

1. Susan A. LaRocca and Denise F. Polit, "Women's Knowledge About the Menopause," *Nursing Research*, vol. 29, no. 1 (Jan.–Feb. 1980), pp. 10–13.

2. Robert A. Wilson, *Feminine Forever* (New York: M. Evans and Co., Inc., 1966).

3. Kathleen I. MacPherson, "Menopause as Disease: The Social Construction of a Metaphor," *ANS/Women's Health*, 1981, pp. 95–113.

4. Ibid.

5. A. A. Haspels and P. A. Van Keep, "Endocrinology and Management of the Peri-Menopause," *Psychosomatics in Peri-Menopause*, ed. A. A. Haspels and H. Musaph (Baltimore: 1979), pp. 57–71.

6. Wulf H. Utian, *Menopause in Modern Perspective*, (New York: Appleton-Century-Crofts, 1980).

7. Clare D. Edman, "The Climacteric," *The Menopause*, ed. Herbert J. Buchsbaum (New York: Springer Verlag, 1983), pp. 23–33.

8. Howard L. Judd et al., "Estrogen Replacement Therapy," *Obstetrics and Gynecology*, vol. 58, No. 3 (Sept. 1981), pp. 267–275.

9. Isaac Schiff et al., "Effects of Estrogen on Sleep and Psychological State of Hypogonadal Women," *Journal of the American Medical Association*, vol. 242, no. 22 (Nov. 30, 1979), pp. 2405–2407.

10. Judd et al., pp. 267–275.

11. Utian, *Menopause.*

12. World Health Organization, "Research on the Menopause," *The Lancet*, vol. 2, no. 8290 (July 17, 1982), pp. 137–138.

13. Council on Scientific Affairs, "Estrogen Replacement in the Menopause," *Journal of the American Medical Association*, vol. 227, no. 1379 (Jan. 21, 1983), pp. 359–361.

14. Utian, *Menopause.*

15. Barbara Gastel and Annabel Hecht, "Estrogens: Another Riddle for Middle Age," *FDA Consumer*, Nov. 1980, HHS Publication No. (FDA) 81-3114.

16. "Researchers Warn on Estrogen Use," *Democrat and Chronicle* (Rochester, N.Y., Oct 17, 1985), p. 3A.

17. R. Don Gambrell, Jr., "Do Hormones Promote or Protect Against Cancer of the Uterus and Breast?" *Menopause Update*, vol. 1, no. 2 (1983), pp. 7–12.

18. Council on Scientific Affairs, "Estrogen Replacement," pp. 359–361.

19. R. Don Gambrell, Jr., "Clinical Use of Progestins in the Menopausal Patient: Dosage and Duration," *The Journal of Reproductive Medicine*, vol. 27, no. 8 (Aug. 1982), pp. 531–538.

20. Utian, *Menopause.*

21. Judd et al., pp. 267–275.

22. Lila E. Nachtigall, "Hormone Therapy: Benefits Versus Risks," *Midlife Wellness*, vol. 1, no. 3 (1983), pp. 29–37.

23. Gambrell, "Clinical Use of Progestins," pp. 531–538.

24. Diana B. Petitti, "Menopausal Estrogens and Vascular Diseases," *Midlife Wellness*, vol. 1, no. 3 (1983), pp. 9–12.

25. Edman, pp. 23–33.

26. Nachtigall, pp. 29–37.

27. Morris Notelovitz, "Estrogen, Lipids and Coronary Heart Disease—A Hypothesis," *Midlife Wellness*, vol. 1, no. 3 (1983), pp. 38–41.

28. Edman, pp. 23–33.

29. Michael R. Soules and William J. Bremner, "The Menopause and Climacteric: Endocrinologic Basis and Associated Symptomology," *Journal of the American Geriatrics Society*, vol. 30, no. 9 (Sept. 1982), pp. 547–561.

30. Notelovitz, "A Hypothesis," pp. 38–41.

31. Petitti, pp. 9–12.

32. Regine Sitruk-Ware, "Newer and Alternative Methods of Hormone Administration," *Midlife Wellness*, vol. 1, no. 3 (1983), pp. 13–17.

33. Utian, *Menopause.*

34. Judd et al., pp. 267–275.

35. World Health Organization, pp. 137–138.

36. *Medical World News* "Workshop Findings Inconclusive on Estrogen, CHD Link," Nov. 14, 1983, pp. 22–23.

37. Nachtigall, pp. 29–37.

38. *Medical World News* "Estrogen, CHD Link," pp. 22–23.

39. *Physician's Desk Reference 1984*, Medical Economics Co. Inc. (Oradell, N.J., 1984).

40. Barbara Seaman and Gideon Seaman, *Women and the Crisis in Sex Hormones* (New York: Bantam Books, 1977).

41. Department of Health, Education and Welfare, "To Be or Not to Be An Estrogen User? Summary of Conclusions of the NIH Consensus Development Conference on Estrogen Use and Postmenopausal Women" (Bethesda, Md., Sept. 13–14, 1979).

42. Ibid.

43. Morris Notelovitz, "Menopause: When to Treat," *Menopause Update*, vol. 1, no. 2 (1983), pp. 27–31.

44. *Physician's Desk Reference 1984*.

45. Gastel and Hecht, HHS Publication No. (FDA) 81-3114.

46. *Physician's Desk Reference 1984*.

47. *Menopause Update*, Research Briefs: "Continuous Treatment With Hormones for Climacteric Complaints," vol. 1, no. 1 (Fall 1982), p. 36; and "Vaginal Estrogen Cream Usage and Its Absorption," vol. 1, no. 2 (1983), p. 47.

48. Notelovitz, "When to Treat," pp. 27- 31.

49. Judd et al., pp. 267–275.

50. *Menopause Update*, "Continuous Treatment," p. 36, and "Vaginal Estrogen Cream," p. 47.

51. Notelovitz et al., "Forum Highlights: Menopause, Role of Hormone Therapy (Part I: Hormone Replacement)," *The Female Patient*, vol. 8 (July 1983), pp. 50/28-40/41.

52. Ibid.

53. Sitruk-Ware, pp. 13–17.

54. Paul G. Stumpf, "The Estradiol Vaginal Ring," *Midlife Wellness*, vol. 1, no. 3 (1983), pp. 21–23.

55. Sitruk-Ware, pp. 13–17.

56. Winnifred B. Cutler, Celso-Ramon García and A. David Edwards, *Menopause: A Guide for Women and the Men Who Love Them* (New York: W. W. Norton & Company, 1983).

57. Stumpf, pp. 21–23.

58. Jean Coope, "Problems Around the Menopause," *The Practitioner*, vol. 227, no. 1379 (May 1983), pp. 793–803.

59. Council on Scientific Affairs, pp. 359–361.

60. Gastel and Hecht, HHS Publication No. (FDA) 81-3114.

61. World Health Organization, pp. 137–138.

62. Utian, *Menopause*.

63. Ibid.

64. Seymour Diamond and Judi Diamond-Falk, *Advice From the Diamond Headache Clinic* (New York: International Universities Press, Inc., 1982).

Chapter 7
Eating Right

1. Olivia Enneking-Ivey, "Needs of the Postmenopausal Woman," *Midlife Wellness*, vol. 1, no. 4 (1984), pp. 2–12.

2. Louisa Rose, ed., *The Menopause Book* (New York: Hawthorn Books Inc., 1977).

3. Frederick J. Stare and Elizabeth M. Whelan, "Nutrition," *Better Homes and Gardens Woman's Health and Medical Guide* (Des Moines, Iowa: Meredith Corp., 1981).

4. National Dairy Council, "The Role of Calcium In Health," *Dairy Council Digest*, vol. 55, no. 1 (Jan./Feb. 1984), pp. 1–8.

5. National Institute on Aging, "Age Page/Osteoporosis: The Bone Thinner" (U.S. Government Printing Office, Dec. 1983), pp. 418–430.

6. Annette Natow and Jo-Ann Heslin, *Nutrition for the Prime of Your Life* (New York: McGraw-Hill, 1983).

7. National Dairy Council, pp. 1 8.

8. National Institute on Aging, pp. 418–430.

9. *Consumer Reports*, "Osteoporosis," Oct. 1984, pp. 576 580.

10. National Dairy Council, pp. 1–8.

11. *Consumer Reports*, "Osteoporosis."

12. Morris Notelovitz and Marsha Ware, *Stand Tall! The Informed Woman's Guide to Preventing Osteoporosis* (Gainesville, Fla.: Triad Publishing Co., 1982).

13. Jane Porcino, *Growing Older, Getting Better* (Addison-Wesley Publishing Co., 1983).

14. Barbara Seaman and Gideon Seaman, *Women and the Crisis in Sex Hormones* (New York: Bantam Books, 1977).

15. Ronald V. Norris and Colleen Sullivan, *PMS· Premenstrual Syndrome* (New York: Rawson Associates, 1983).

16. "Salt: How Much Is Too Much?" *Menopause Update*, vol. 1, no. 1 (Fall 1982), pp. 28–32.

17. National Dairy Council, "Diet, Nutrition and Cancer," *Dairy Council Digest*, vol. 54, no. 6 (Nov./Dec. 1983) pp. 31–36.

18. *Menopause Update*, "Salt," pp. 28–32.

19. U.S. Department of Agriculture, U.S. Dept. of Health and Human Services, "Sodium."

20. H. Holly Shimizu, "Do Yourself a Flavor," *FDA Consumer*, reprinted from April 1984, HHS Publication No. (FDA) 84-2192.

21. "Zinc Deficiency May Result From Long-Term Use of Diuretics," *Menopause Update*, vol. 1, no. 2 (1983), p. 45.

22. American Medical Association, "Personal Health Care," *Newsweek*, special advertising supplement, Nov, 7, 1983.

23. U.S. Department of Health and Human Services, National Institutes of Health, *Cancer Prevention*, NIH Publication No. 84-2671 (Feb. 1984).

24. John A. Baron, "Smoking and Estrogen-Related Disease," *American Journal of Epidemiology*, vol. 119, no. 1 (1984), pp. 9–21.

25. Ilene Singer Levinson, "Research Briefs: Menopause, Smoking and Tooth Loss," *Midlife Wellness*, vol. 1, no. 3 (1983), p. 45.

26. Baron, pp. 9–21.

27. American Medical Association, "Health Care."

28. Jane Brody, *Jane Brody's Nutrition Book* (New York: W. W. Norton & Co., 1981).

29. Barbara Harland and Annabel Hecht, "Grandma Called It Roughage," *FDA Consumer*, reprinted from July–Aug. 1977, HHS Publication No. (FDA) 78-2087.

30. National Dairy Council, "Diet, Nutrition and Cancer," pp. 31–36.

31. Lisa Reimer, "Nutrition and Cancer–A Brief Overview," *Midlife Wellness*, vol. 1, no. 4 (1984), pp. 13–19.

32. Brody, *Nutrition Book*.

33. Harland and Hecht, "Roughage," 78-2087.

34. Brody, *Nutrition Book*.

35. National Dairy Council, "Diet, Nutrition and Cancer," pp. 31–36.

36. Reimer, pp. 13–19.

37. Ibid.

38. American Institute for Cancer Research, *Dietary Guidelines to Lower Cancer Risk*, June 1982.

39. National Dairy Council, "Diet, Nutrition and Cancer," pp. 31–36.

40. Reimer, pp. 13–19.

Chapter 8
Exercise: The Best Anti-Aging Pill

1. American Medical Association, *The American Medical Association Guide to Health and Well-Being After 50* (New York: Random House, 1984).

2. Mona M. Shangold, "Sports and Exercise," *The Menopause*, ed. Herbert J. Buchsbaum (New York: Springer Verlag, 1983), pp. 199–203.

3. Christian W. Zauner, "Exercise: A Health Care Need," *Midlife Wellness*, vol. 1, no. 4 (1984), pp. 33–43.

4. American Medical Association, *Health and Well-Being After 50*.

5. Julia Klein, "Running Away from Depression," *Ms.*, May 1983, pp. 85–88.

6. Jane Porcino, *Growing Older, Getting Better* (Addison-Wesley Publishing Co., 1983).

7. Shangold, pp. 199–203.

8. Christine A. Gregory, "Possible Influence of Physical Activity on Musculo-skeletal Symptoms of Menopausal and Postmenopausal Women," *JOGN Nursing*, Mar./Apr. 1982, pp. 103–107.

9. American Heart Association Publications, *Walking for a Healthy Heart*, 1984.

10. Zauner, pp. 33–43.

11. American Heart Association Publications, *Walking*.

12. American Medical Association, "Special Advertising Supplement," *Newsweek*, Nov. 7, 1983.

13. Charles Kuntzleman, *The Exerciser's Handbook* (New York: David McKay Co., 1978).

14. National Dairy Council, *What to Know About a Weight-Control Diet Before You Eat One*, 1981.

15. Olivia Enneking-Ivey, "Needs of the Postmenopausal Woman," *Midlife Wellness*, vol. 1, no. 4 (1984), pp. 2–12.

16. "Warning: Fat, Smoke Can Kill," *Democrat and Chronicle* (Rochester, N.Y., Feb. 14, 1985), p. 1 and 15 A.

17. National Dairy Council, *What to Know About a Weight-Control Diet*.

18. Ibid.

Chapter 9
Sexuality

1. Edward M. Brecher, *Love, Sex and Aging: A Consumers Union Report* (Boston: Little, Brown & Co., 1984)

2. Shere Hite, *The Hite Report* (New York: Macmillan Publishing Co., 1976).

3. Alfred C. Kinsey et al., *Sexual Behavior in the Human Female* (W. B. Saunders Company, 1953).

4. William H. Masters and Virginia E. Johnson, *Human Sexual Inadequacy* (Boston: Little, Brown & Co., 1970).

5. William H. Masters and Virginia E. Johnson, *Human Sexual Response* (Boston: Little, Brown & Co., 1966).

6. Hite, *Hite Report*.

7. Bernard D. Starr and Marcella B. Weiner, *The Starr-Weiner Report on Sex and Sexuality in the Mature Years* (New York: Stein and Day, 1981).

8. Lorraine Dennerstein et al., "Hormones and Sexuality: Effect of Estrogen and Progestogen," *Obstetrics and Gynecology*, vol. 56, no. 3 (Sept. 1980), pp. 316–322.

9. Paula Weideger, *Menstruation and Menopause* (New York: Alfred A. Knopf, 1976).

10. Martha J. Morell et al., "The Influence of Age and Cycling Status on Sexual Arousability in Women," *American Journal of Obstetrics and Gynecology*, vol. 148, no. 1 (Jan. 1, 1984), pp. 66–71.

11. Wulf H. Utian, *Menopause in Modern Perspective* (New York: Appleton-Century-Crofts, 1980).

12. Wulf H. Utian, "Vaginal Function in Postmenopausal Women," letter, *Journal of the American Medical Association*, vol. 249, no. 2 (Jan. 14, 1983), pp. 194–195.

13. Sheila E. Dreisen, "The Sexually Active Middle Adult," *American Journal of Nursing*, vol. 75, no. 5 (June 1975), pp. 1001–1004.

14. Masters, *Sexual Inadequacy*.

15. Masters, *Sexual Response*.

16. Ibid.

17. James P. Semmens, "Sexuality," *The Menopause*, ed. Herbert J. Buchsbaum (New York: Springer Verlag, 1983), pp. 175–180.

18. Rosetta Reitz, *Menopause: A Positive Approach* (Radnor, Pa.: Chilton Book Co., 1977).

19. Maggie Lettvin, *Maggie's Woman's Book* (New York: Houghton Mifflin Co., 1980).

20. Leon Zussman et al., "Sexual Response After Hyst-oophorectomy: Recent Studies and Reconsideration of Psychogenesis," *American Journal of Obstetrics and Gynecology*, vol. 140, no. 7 (Aug. 1, 1981), pp. 725–729.

21. Charles W. Lloyd, "Sexuality in the Climacteric," *The Menopause: Comprehensive Management* (Masson Pub., Inc., 1980), pp. 101–110.

22. Susanne Morgan, *Coping With a Hysterectomy* (New York: The Dial Press, 1982).

23. Zussman and Zussman, Sunley, and Bjornson, pp. 725–729.

24. Semmens, pp. 445–448.

25. Masters, *Sexual Response*.

26. Roslyn Cutick, "Special Needs of Perimenopausal Women," *JOGN Nursing (Supplement)*, Mar./Apr. 1984, pp. 68s–73s.

27. Boston Women's Health Book Collective, *The New Our Bodies, Ourselves* (New York: Simon & Schuster, 1984).

28. Masters, *Sexual Response*.

29. Boston Women's Health Book Collective.

30. Lynda Maduras and Jane Patterson, *Womancare* (New York: Avon Books, 1981).

31. Gail Sheehy, *Passages* (New York: E. P. Dutton & Co., Inc., 1976).

32. Masters, *Sexual Response*.

33. Dreisen, pp. 1001–1004.

34. *Time*, "Is Male Menopause A Myth?" Vol. 114, no. 8 (Aug. 20, 1979), p. 68.

35. American Medical Association, *The American Medical Association Guide to Health and Well-Being After 50* (New York: Random House, 1984).

36. National Institute on Aging, "Age Page: Sexuality in Later Life," Oct. 1981.

37. Semmens, pp. 175–180.

38. American Medical Association, *Health and Well-Being After 50*.

Chapter 10
Body Changes

1. James L. Breen, "Woman's Health: Pelvic Relaxation" (press release from the American College of Obstetricians and Gynecologists, Sept. 12, 1983).

2. Ibid.

3. Wulf H. Utian, *Menopause in Modern Perspective* (New York: Appleton-Century-Crofts, 1980).

4. Harold Hopkins, "Tan Now, Pay Later?" *FDA Consumer*, reprinted from April 1982, HHS Publication (FDA) 82-1095.

5. American Medical Association, *The AMA Book of Skin and Hair Care*, ed., Linda Allen Schoen (New York: J. B. Lippincott Co., 1976).

6. William Dvorine, *A Dermatologist's Guide to Home Skin Treatment* (New York: Charles Scribner's Sons, 1983).

7. Candace Lyle Hogan, "How to Keep Your Skin Fit," *Ms.*, May 1984, p. 127.

8. American Academy of Dermatology, "Aging of the Skin," information sheet distributed 1984.

9. *Consumer Reports*, "Fade Creams," vol. 50, no. 1 (Jan., 1985), p. 12.

10. Arnold W. Klein, James H. Sternberg and Paul Bernstein, *The Skin Book* (New York: Macmillan Publishing Co., 1980).

11. Deborah Blumenthal, "Coping With Unwanted Hair," *New York Times Magazine*, May 22, 1983, p. 71.

12. Ibid.

13. American Medical Association, *The American Medical Association Guide to Health and Well-Being After 50* (New York: Random House, 1984).

14. Harry W. Danelli, "Postmenopausal Tooth Loss," *Archives of Internal Medicine*, vol. 143, no. 9 (Sept. 1983), pp. 1678–1682.

15. Ibid.

16. Ibid.

17. Ibid.

18. Jane Porcino, *Growing Older, Getting Better* (Addison-Wesley Publishing Co., 1983).

19. American Academy of Opthalmology publications, *Glaucoma: It Can Take Your Sight Away*, 1984.

20. American Academy of Opthalmology publications, *Diabetic Retinopathy*, 1984.

Chapter 11
Osteoporosis

1. Charles Y. C. Pak, "Postmenopausal Osteoporosis," *The Menopause*, ed. Herbert J. Buchsbaum (New York: Springer Verlag, 1983), pp. 35–54.

2. "Osteoporosis, The 'Silent' Disease, Strikes One in Four Women Over 65, An Expert Warns," *People*, April 1, 1985, p. 129.

3. Clare D. Edman, "The Climacteric," *The Menopause*, ed. Herbert J. Buchsbaum (New York: Springer Verlag, 1983), pp. 23–33.

4. Libby Machol, "Postmenopausal Osteoporosis: New Approaches to Prevention," *Contemporary Ob/Gyn*, vol. 20 (Aug. 1982), pp. 153–161.

5. B. E. Christopher Nordon, "Bone Loss at the Menopause," *Menopause Update*, vol. 1, no. 1 (Fall, 1982), pp. 5–9.

6. Wulf H. Utian, *Menopause in Modern Perspective* (New York: Appleton-Century-Crofts, 1980).

7. *Consumer Reports*, "Osteoporosis," Oct. 1984, pp. 576–580.

8. Edman, pp. 23–33.

9. Utian, *Modern Perspective*.

10. The American College of Obstetricians and Gynecologists, *ACOG Technical Bulletin*, no. 72 (October 1983).

11. Ranney Brooks, "Woman's Health: Osteoporosis," ACOG News Release, Sept. 27, 1982.

12. *Consumer Reports*, pp. 576–580.

13. Morris Notelovitz and Marsha Ware, *Stand Tall! The Informed Woman's Guide to Preventing Osteoporosis* (Gainesville, Fla.: Triad Publishing Co., 1982).

14. Edman, pp. 23–33.

15. Notelovitz and Ware, *Stand Tall!*

16. Ibid.

17. Christine A. Gregory, "Possible Influence of Physical Activity on Musculo-Skeletal Symptoms of Menopausal and Postmenopausal Women," *JOGN Nursing*, Mar./Apr. 1982, pp. 103–107.

18. *Consumer Reports*, pp. 576–580.

19. National Dairy Council, *Are You at Risk for Bone Disease?* 1984.

20. National Dairy Council, "The Role of Calcium in Health," *Dairy Council Digest*, vol. 55, no. 1 (Jan./Feb. 1984), pp. 1–8.

21. Notelovitz and Ware, *Stand Tall!*

22. Ibid.

23. "Osteoporosis, 'The Silent Disease,'" p. 129.

24. "Thyroid Supplements May Decrease Bone Mass," *Menopause Update*, p. 35.

25. National Dairy Council, "The Role of Calcium," pp. 1–8.

26. Utian, *Modern Perspective*.

27. Ilene Singer Levinson, "Thiazide Diuretics and Bone Mineral Content," *Midlife Wellness*, vol. 1, no. 3 (1983), pp. 44–45.

28. Notelovitz and Ware, *Stand Tall!*

29. *Consumer Reports*, pp. 576–580.

30. CCS News, "Bone Densometer—Measuring Bone Mineral Content in the Forearm," and "Dual-Photon Body Scanning—Measuring Total Body Bone Mineral," *Menopause Update*, vol. 1, no. 2 (1983), p. 54.

31. Ilene Singer Levinson, "Research Briefs: A New Blood Test for Osteoporosis?" *Midlife Wellness*, vol. 1, no. 4 (1984), p. 55.

32. National Dairy Council, "The Role of Calcium," pp. 1–8.

33. *Consumer Reports*, pp. 576–580.

34. "Osteoporosis, 'The Silent Disease,'" p. 129.

35. *Menopause Update*, "Premature Bone Loss in Non-Menstruating Women," vol. 1, no. 1 (Fall 1982), p. 35.

36. Notelovitz and Ware, *Stand Tall!*

37. National Dairy Council, "The Role of Calcium," pp. 1–8.

38. Malcolm I. Whitehead, "Long-Term Usage of Hormones . . . Is It Beneficial in Preventing Postmenopausal Osteoporosis?" *Midlife Wellness*, vol. 1, no. 3 (1983), pp. 2–8.

39. Utian, *Modern Perspective*.

40. Whitehead, pp. 2–8.

41. Leah J. Roen, "Environmental Variables Influencing Osteoporosis," *Midlife Wellness*, vol. 1, no. 3 (1983), pp. 51–55.

42. National Institutes of Health, U.S. Department of Health and Human Services, "Osteoporosis, Cause, Treatment, Prevention," April 1983.

43. Levinson, "Thiazide Diuretics and Bone Mineral Content," pp. 44–45.

Chapter 12
Staying Healthy: A Gynecologic Guide

1. Genevieve Fitzpatrick, "Caring for the Patient with Cancer of the Cervix," *Nursing Care*, vol. 9, no. 1, American Cancer Society, Inc., 1976.

2. Felicia Stewart et al., *My Body My Health* (New York: John Wiley & Sons, 1979).

3. American Cancer Society, *1985 Cancer Facts and Figures*.

4. Bruce Shephard and Carol Shephard, *The Complete Guide to Women's Health* (Tampa, Fla.: Mariner Publishing Co., 1982).

5. Boston Women's Health Book Collective, *The New Our Bodies, Our selves* (New York: Simon & Schuster, 1984).

6. Norma Swenson, "Breast Cancer. The Problem," *Breast Cancer—Resource Guide I* (Washington, D.C.: National Women's Health Network, 1981).

7. American Cancer Society, *Facts and Figures*.

8. Boston Women's Health Book Collective, *The New Our Bodies, Ourselves*.

9. Maryann Napoli, "Breast Cancer: The Truth About Early Detection," *Ms.*, May 1983, pp. 86–89.

10. American Institute for Cancer Research, *Questions and Answers About Breast Lumps*, distributed 1984.

11. Wende Logan, "Questions I Always Wanted to Ask—But Didn't," *Midlife Wellness*, vol. 2, no. 2 (1985), pp. 85–87.

12. Bernard Fisher et al., "Five Year Results of a Randomized Clinical Trial Comparing Total Mastectomy and Segmental Mastectomy With or Without Radiation in the Treatment of Breast Cancer," *The New England Journal of Medicine*, vol. 312, no. 11 (Mar. 14, 1985), pp. 666–673.

13. "Cancer: A Radical Departure," *Newsweek*, Mar. 25, 1985, p. 91.

14. Swenson, "Breast Cancer."

15. Daniel E. Kenady, "Fibrocystic Disease of the Breast," *Midlife Wellness*, vol. 2, no. 2 (1985), pp. 73–78.

16. Boston Women's Health Book Collective.

17. *McCall's*, "When Breast Lumps Aren't Cancer," May 1985, pp. 65–66.

18. Arlene Weinshelbaum and Edward Weinshelbaum, "Mammography," *Midlife Wellness*, vol. 2, no. 2 (1985), pp. 98–102.

19. National Cancer Institute, "Breast Cancer: We're Making Progress Every Day," NIH Publication No. 83–2409, 1983.

20. Napoli, pp. 86–89.

21. William N. Spellacy, "Abnormal Bleeding," *Clinical Obstetrics and Gynecology*, vol. 26, no. 3 (Sept. 1983), pp. 702–707.

22. David R. Meldrum, "Perimenopausal Menstrual Problems," *Clinical Obstetrics and Gynecology*, vol. 26, no. 3 (Sept. 1983), pp. 762–768.

23. Herbert H. Keyser, *Women Under the Knife* (Philadelphia: George F. Stickley Co., 1984).

24. Lynda Madaras and Jane Patterson, *Womancare* (New York: Avon Books, 1981).

25. Keyser, *Women Under the Knife.*

26. Boston Women's Health Book Collective.

27. Charles L. Easterday, David A. Grimes and Joseph A. Riggs, "Hysterectomy in the United States," *Obstetrics and Gynecology*, vol. 62, no. 2 (Aug. 1983), pp. 203–212.

28. Leon Zussman et al., "Sexual Response After Hyst-Oophorectomy: Recent Studies and Reconsideration of Psychogenesis," *American Journal of Obstetrics and Gynecology*, vol. 140, no. 7 (Aug. 1, 1981), pp. 725–729.

29. Boston Women's Health Book Collective.

30. Easterday, Grimes and Riggs, pp. 203–212.

31. Ibid.

32. Ibid.

Bibliography

Abarbanel, Karin, and Siegel, Connie MoClung. *Woman's Work Book*. New York: Praeger Publishers, 1975.

Alington-MacKinnon, Diane, and Troll, Lillian E. "The Adaptive Function of the Menopause: A Devil's Advocate Position." *Journal of the American Geriatrics Society*, vol. 29, no. 8, Aug. 1981:349–353.

Aloia, John F., Cohn, Stanton H., Vaswani, Ashok, Yeh, James K., Yuen, Kapo, and Ellis, Kenneth. "Risk Factors for Postmenopausal Osteoporosis." The American Journal of Medicine, vol. 78, no. 1, Jan. 1985:95–100.

American Academy of Dermatology. "Aging of the Skin." Information sheet distributed 1984.

American Academy of Facial Plastic and Reconstructive Surgery publications. *Facts About Facelift Surgery*, 1984.

——. *Facts About Plastic Surgery of the Eyelid and Eyebrow*, 1984.

——. *Plastic Surgery*, 1984.

The American Brittle Bone Society. "Osteoporosis: Cause and Effect," 1984.

American Academy of Opthalmology publications. *Cataract: Clouding of the Lens of Sight*, 1984.

——. *Diabetic Retinopathy*, 1984.

——. *Glaucoma: It Can Take Your Sight Away*, 1984.

——. *Seeing Well As You Grow Older*, 1984.

American Cancer Society. *(BSE) Not for Women Only*, 1984

——. *1985 Cancer Facts and Figures*.

——. *Mammography 1982: A Statement of the American Cancer Society*.

American College of Obstetricians and Gynecologists. "A Postmenopausal Regimen May Cut Risk of Breast Cancer." *1983 ACOG Annual*.

——. *ACOG Technical Bulletin*, no. 70, June 1983.

——. *ACOG Technical* Bulletin, no. 72, Oct. 1983.

——. "Sex and the Senior Citizen." Press release, June 14, 1982.

American Heart Association publications. *Cholesterol and Your Heart*, 1984.

——. *Eat Well But Eat Wisely*, 1981.

——. *How You Can Help Your Doctor Treat High Blood Pressure*, 1984.

——. *Piecing Together the Sodium Puzzle*, 1984.

——. *Salt, Sodium and Blood Pressure*, 1984.

American Institute for Cancer Research. *Dietary Guidelines to Lower Cancer Risk*, June 1982.

——. *Questions and Answers About Breast Lumps*, distributed 1984.

——. *American Institute for Cancer Research Newsletter*. "Fat and Cancer: How Fat in Diet Affects Cancer Risk," Fall 1984:2–3.

——. "Keep in Touch With Yourself," Issue 3, Spring 1984.

American Medical Association. *The AMA Book of Skin and Hair Care*. Edited by Linda Allen Schoen. New York: J. B. Lippincott Co., 1976.

——. *The AMA Guide to Health and Well-Being After 50*. New York: Random House, Inc., 1984.

——. "Personal Health Care." Special supplement in *Newsweek*, Oct. 29, 1984.

——. Special advertising supplement in *Newsweek*, Nov. 7, 1983.

Anderson, F. S., Transbol, I., and Christiansen, C. "Is Cigarette Smoking a Promoter of the Menopause?" *Acta Med. Scand.*, vol. 212, no. 3, 1982:137–139.

Archer, David. "Biomedical Findings and Medical Management of the Menopause." *Changing Perspectives on Menopause*. Edited by A. Voda, M. Dinnerstein, and S. O'Donnell. Austin: University of Texas Press, 1982.

Armitage, Karen J., Schneiderman, Lawrence J., and Bass, Robert A. "Response of Physicians to Medical Complaints in Men and Women." *Journal of the American Medical Association*, vol. 241, no. 20, May 18, 1979:2186–2187.

Bachmann, Gloria A. "Sexual Response and Hormone Therapy." *Menopause Update*, vol. 1, no. 2, 1983:23–26.

Baran, John A. "Smoking and Estrogen-Related Disease." *American Journal of Epidemiology*, vol. 119, no. 1, 1984:9–21.

Bates, William G. "On the Nature of the Hot Flash." *Clinical Obstetrics and Gynecology*, vol. 24, no. 1, March 1981:231–241.

Benson, Herbert. *The Relaxation Response.* New York: William Morrow & Co., 1975.

——, with Proctor, William. "Beating Illness with the Faith Factor." *Prevention*, vol. 36, no. 5, May 1984:24–32.

Blumenthal, Deborah. "Coping With Unwanted Hair." *New York Times Magazine*, May 22, 1983:71.

——. "The Often Elusive Pursuit of Sleep." *The New York Times Magazine*, Dec. 11, 1983:24.

Bolles, Richard Nelson. *What Color Is Your Parachute?* Berkeley, Calif: Ten Speed Press, 1983.

Boston Women's Health Book Collective. *Our Bodies, Ourselves.* New York: Simon & Schuster, 1976.

——. *The New Our Bodies, Ourselves.* New York: Simon & Schuster, 1984.

Brand, Pam. "A Henna Headtrip." *Ms.*, May 1983:45–48.

Brecher, Edward M. *Love, Sex and Aging: A Consumers Union Report.* Boston: Little, Brown & Co., 1984.

Ditch, James L. "The Help of Estrogen." The American College of Obstetricians and Gynecologists. News release, Dec. 5, 1983.

——. "Sex After 50." News release from The American College of Obstetricians and Gynecologists, Sept. 26, 1983.

——. "What Was, What Is and What May Be." President Address at the 31st Annual Clinical Meeting of the American College of Obstetricians and Gynecologists, Atlanta, Georgia, May 11, 1983.

——. "Woman's Health: Pelvic Relaxation." Press release from the American College of Obstetricians and Gynecologists, Sept. 12, 1983.

Brincat, M., Moniz, C. F., Studd, J. W. W., Darby, A. J., Magos, A. and Cooper, D. "Sex Hormones and Skin Collagen Content in Postmenopausal Women." *British Medical Journal*, vol. 287, no. 6402, Nov. 5, 1983:1337–38.

Brody, Jane. *Jane Brody's Nutrition Book.* New York: W. W. Norton & Co., 1981.

——. "Personal Health/For Many Men, Midlife Is a Crucial Turning Point. . ." *The New York Times*, July 22, 1981:C-8.

Brooks, Ranney. "Woman's Health: Osteoporosis." ACOG news release, Sept. 27, 1982.

Bungay, G. T., Vessey, M. P., and McPherson, C. K. "Study of Symptoms in Middle Life With Special Reference to the Menopause." *British Medical Journal*, vol. 281, no. 6233, July 19, 1980:181–183.

Caldwell, Laura Ryan. "Questions and Answers About the Menopause." *American Journal of Nursing*, vol. 82, no. 7, July 1982:1100.

Casper, R. F., Yen, S. S. C., and Wilkes, M. M. "Menopausal Flushes: A Neuroendocrine Link with Pulsatile Luteinizing Hormone Secretion." *Science*, vol. 205, Aug. 24, 1979:823–825.

CCS News. "Bone Densometer—Measuring Bone Mineral Content in the Forearm," and "Dual-Photon Body Scanning—Measuring Total Body Bone Mineral." *Menopause Update*, vol. 1, no. 2, 1983:54.

Clay, Vidal S. "Menopause." *Better Homes and Gardens Woman's Health and Medical Guide.* Edited by Patricia J. Cooper. Des Moines: Meredith Corporation, 1981:312–318.

Connell, Elizabeth. "Contraceptive Needs of the Middle Years." *Menopause Update,* vol. 1, no. 2, 1983:34–37.

Consumer Reports. "Fade Creams," vol. 50, no. 1, Jan. 1985:12.

———. "Osteoporosis," Oct. 1984:576–580.

Consumers Union. "Caffeine: How to Consume Less." *Consumer Reports,* vol. 46, no. 10, Oct. 1981:597–599.

Coope, Jean. "Problems Around the Menopause." *The Practitioner,* vol. 227, no. 1379, May 1983:793–803.

———. "Symptoms in Middle Life and the Menopause," letter. *British Medical* Journal, vol. 281, no. 243, 1980:811.

Cope, E. "Physical Changes Associated with the Post-Menopausal Years." *The Management of The Menopause and Post-Menopausal Years.* Edited by Stuart Campbell. Baltimore: University Park Press, 1976:29–42.

Corbett, Louise. "Getting Our Bodies Back: Menopause Self-Help Groups." Information sheet from The Menopause Collective, Cambridge, Mass., 1981.

Council on Scientific Affairs. "Council Report: Estrogen Replacement in the Menopause." *Journal of the American Medical Association,* vol. 249, no. 3, Jan 21, 1983:359–361.

Court, W. E. "Ginseng—A Chinese Folk Medicine of Current Interest." *The Pharmaceutical Journal,* Mar. 1, 1975:180–181.

Cutick, Roslyn. "Special Needs of Perimenopausal and Menopausal Women." *JOGN Nursing (Supplement),* Mar./Apr. 1984:68s–73s.

Cutler, Winnifred B., García, Celso-Ramon, and Edwards, David, A. *Menopause: A Guide for Women and the Men Who Love Them.* New York: W. W. Norton & Company, 1983.

Danelli, Harry W. "Postmenopausal Tooth Loss." *Archives of Internal Medicine,* vol. 143, no. 9, Sept. 1983:1678–82.

Davis, Edward M., and Meilach, Dona Z. *A Doctor Discusses Menopause and Estrogens.* Chicago: Budlong Press Co., 1981.

Democrat and Chronicle. "Sex Hormones Help Predict Recurrence of Breast Cancer," Rochester, N.Y., Dec. 1, 1983:8A.

———. "Warning: Fat, Smoke Can Kill," Rochester, N.Y., Feb. 14, 1985:1/ 15A.

———. "Research Warns on Estrogen Use," Rochester, N.Y., Oct. 17, 1985:8A.

Dennerstein, Lorraine, Burrows, Graham D., Wood, Carl, and Graeme, Hyman. "Hormones and Sexuality: Effect of Estrogen and Progestogen." *Obstetrics and Gynecology,* vol. 56, no. 3, Sept. 1980:316–322.

De Vane, Gary. "Hormonal Changes During the Climacteric." *Menopause Update,* vol. 1, no. 2, 1983:2–6.

De Vries, Herbert A. with Hales, Dianne. *Fitness After Fifty.* New York: Charles Scribner's Sons, 1982.

Dewhurst, C. J. "Frequency and Severity of Menopausal Symptoms." *The Management of the Menopause and Post-Menopausal Years.* Edited by Stuart Campbell. Baltimore: University Park Press, 1976:25–27.

Dewhurst, Sir John. "Postmenopausal Bleeding from Benign Causes." *Clinical Obstetrics and Gynecology*, vol. 26, no. 3, Sept. 1983:769–776.

Diamond, Seymour and Diamond-Falk, Judi. *Advice from the Diamond Headache Clinic.* New York: International Universities Press, Inc. 1982.

Diekelmann, Nancy. "Emotional Tasks of the Middle Adult." *American Journal of Nursing*, vol. 75, no. 6, June 1975:997–1001.

Diekelman, Nancy and Galloway, Karen. "A Time of Change." *American Journal of Nursing*, vol. 75, no. 6, June 1975:994–996.

Dreisen, Sheila E. "The Sexually Active Middle Adult." *American Journal of Nursing*, vol. 75, no. 6, June 1975:1001–04.

Dubinsky, Sue. "Breast Self-Examination: Techniques and Tips." *Midlife Wellness*, vol. 2, no. 2, 1985:88–90.

Dvorine, William. *A Dermatologist's Guide to Home Skin Treatment.* New York: Charles Scribner's Sons, 1983.

Dvrenfurth, Inge. "Endocrine Functions in the Woman's Second Half of Life." *Changing Perspectives on Menopause.* Edited by A. Voda, M. Dinnerstein, and S. R. O'Donnell. Austin: University of Texas Press, 1982:307–334.

Easterday, Charles L., Grimes, David A., and Riggs, Joseph A. "Hysterectomy in the United States." *Obstetrics and Gynecology*, vol. 62, no. 2, Aug. 1983:203–212.

Edelson, Edward. "Menopause and Birth Control." *Woman's Day*, Sept. 1, 1981:6–7.

Edman, Clare, D. "The Climacteric." *The Menopause.* Edited by Herbert J. Buchsbaum. New York: Springer-Verlag, 1983.

Enneking-Ivey, Olivia. "Needs of the Postmenopausal Woman." *Midlife Wellness*, vol. 1, no. 4, 1984:2–12.

Erlik, Yohanan, Meldrum, David R., and Judd, Howard L. "Estrogen Levels in Postmenopausal Women with Hot Flashes." *Obstetrics and Gynecology*, vol. 59, no. 4, April 1982:403–407.

Eye Health Service Commission for the Visually Handicapped. *Eyes Over Forty.* New York State Department of Social Services, brochure, July 1971.

Farrah, Adelaide P. "A Woman's Breasts." *Health*, Aug. 1984:57.

FDA Consumer. "The Latest Caffeine Scorecard," vol. 18, no. 2, March 1984:14–15.

Feibleman, Cary E. "Skin Problems." *Better Homes and Gardens Woman's Health and Medical Guide.* Des Moines, Iowa: Meredith Corp., 1981:560–581.

Feinberg, Herbert S. *All About Hair.* New York: Simon & Schuster, 1979.

Fink, Paul J. "Psychiatric Myths of the Menopause." *The Menopause: Com-

prehensive Management. Edited by Bernard A. Eskin. Masson Pub., USA, 1980:111–128.

Fisher, Bernard, Baver, Madeline, Margolese, Richard et al. "Five Year Results of a Randomized Clinical Trial Comparing Total Mastectomy and Segmental Mastectomy With or Without Radiation in the Treatment of Breast Cancer." *The New England Journal of Medicine*, vol. 312, no. 11, Mar. 14:666–673.

Fitzpatrick, Genevieve. "Caring for the Patient with Cancer of the Cervix." *Nursing Care*, vol. 9, no. 1, 1976. Reprint distributed by the American Cancer Society, Inc.

Flint, Marcha P. "The Menopause: Reward or Punishment?" *Psychosomatics*, vol. 16, Oct/Nov/Dec. 1975:161–163.

———. "Sociocultural Aspects of the Menopause." *Menopause Update*, vol. 1, no. 1, Fall 1982:22–24.

———. "Transcultural Influences in Peri-Menopausal Research." *Psychosomatics in Peri-Menopause*. Edited by A. A. Haspels and H. Musaph. Baltimore: University Park Press, 1979:41–55.

Gambrell, R. Don Jr. "Clinical Use of Progestins in the Menopausal Patient: Dosage and Duration." *The Journal of Reproductive Medicine*, supplement, vol. 27, no. 8, Aug. 1982:531–538.

———. "Do Hormones Promote or Protect Against Cancer of the Uterus and Breast?" *Menopause Update*, vol. 1, no. 2, 1983:7–12.

Gastel, Barbara and Hecht, Annabel. "Estrogens: Another Riddle for Middle Age." *FDA Consumer*. HHS Publication No. (FDA) 81–3114, Nov. 1980.

Gignac, Louis and Warsaw, Jacqueline. *Everything You Need to Know to Have Great Looking Hair*. New York: The Viking Press, 1981.

Good Housekeeping. "How to Get Rid of Unwanted Hair," July 1983:199.

Goodman, Ellen. "Gary Makes Her Feel Young Again." The Boston Globe Newspaper Company/Washington Post Writers Group, March 30, 1984.

Gorrie, Trula Myers. "Postmenopausal Osteoporosis." *JOGN Nursing*, July/Aug. 1982:214–219.

Greenblatt, Robert. "The Menopause—Past, Present and Future." *Menopause Update*, vol. 1, no. 1, Fall 1982:10–14.

Gregory, Christine A. "Possible Influence of Physical Activity on Musculo-Skeletal Symptoms of Menopausal and Postmenopausal Women." *JOGN Nursing*, Mar./Apr. 1982:103–107.

Grossman, John. "Facing an Operation." *McCall's*, Aug. 1984:136–139.

Hahn, Ricardo G., Nachtigall, Robert D., and Davies, Terence C. "Compliance Difficulties with Progestin-Supplemented Estrogen Replacement Therapy." *The Journal of Family Practice*, vol. 18, no. 3, 1984:411–414.

Harland, Barbara and Hecht, Annabel. "Grandma Called It Roughage." *FDA Consumer*. Reprinted from July/Aug. 1977, HHS Publication No. (FDA) 78-2087.

Haspels, A. A. and Van Keep, P. A. "Endocrinology and Management of the Peri-Menopause." *Psychosomatics in Peri-Menopause*. Edited by A. A. Haspels and H. Musaph. Baltimore: University Park Press, 1979:57–71.

Haycock, Christine and Sherman, Gail. "Fitness." *Better Homes and Gardens Woman's Health and Medical Guide*. Des Moines, Iowa: Meredith Corporation, 1981:62–67.

Health. "Stop Aging Skin," vol. 14, no. 2, Feb. 1982:52.

Hemphill, Delores; and Kimber, Yvonne. "A Positive Look at Menopause." *Teacher Training Manual*, Planned Parenthood of Central Missouri, 1982.

Hite, Shere. *The Hite Report*. New York: Macmillan Publishing Co., Inc., 1976.

Hogan, Candace Lyle. "How to Keep Your Skin Fit." *Ms.*, May 1984:127.

Holmes, Thomas H. and Rahe, Richard H. "The Social Readjustment Rating Scale." *Journal of Psychosomatic Research*, vol. 2, no. 2, Aug. 1967:213–218.

Hopkins, Harold. "Tan Now, Pay Later?" *FDA Consumer*. Reprinted from April 1982, HHS Publication (FDA) 82-1095.

Hubbell, Nancy Cooper. "Breasts." *Better Homes and Gardens Woman's Health and Medical Guide*. Des Moines, Iowa: Meredith Corp., 1981:148–160.

Jones, Esther C. "The Post-Fertile Life of Non-Human Primates and Other Mammals." *Psychosomatics in Peri-Menopause*. Edited by A. A. Haspels and H. Musaph. Baltimore: University Park Press, 1979:13–39.

Judd, Howard L., Cleary, Robert E., Creasman, William T., Frgge, David C., Kase, Nathan, Rosenwales, Zev, and Tagatz, George E. "Estrogen Replacement Therapy." *Obstetrics and Gynecology*, vol. 58, no. 3, Sept. 1981:267–275.

Kaufert, Pat and Syrotuik, John. "Symptom Reporting at the Menopause." *Social Science Medicine*, vol. 15 E, 1981:173–184.

Kenady, Daniel E. "Fibrocystic Disease of the Breast." *Midlife Wellness*, vol. 2, no. 2, 1985:73–78.

Keyser, Herbert H. *Women Under the Knife*. Philadelphia: George F. Stickley Co., 1984.

Kinsey, Alfred, C., Pomeroy, Wardell B., Martin, Clyde, E., and Gebhard, Paul H. *Sexual Behavior in the Human Female*. W. B. Saunders Company, 1953.

Klein, Arnold W., Sternberg, James H., and Bernstein, Paul. *The Skin Book*. New York: Macmillan Publishing Co., 1980.

Klein, Julia. "Running Away from Depression. *Ms.*, May, 1983:85–88.

Korenman, Stanley G. "Menopausal Endocrinology and Management." *Archives of Internal Medicine*, vol. 142, June 1982:1131–1136.

Kosch, Shae and Spring, Anita. "Breast Disease and Breast Self-Examination." *Midlife Wellness*, vol. 2, no. 2, 1985:80–84.

Krailo, M. D. and Pike, M. C. "Estimation of the Distribution of Age at Menopause from Prevalence Data." *American Journal of Epidemiology.* vol. 117, no. 3, March 1983.

Kuntzleman, Charles. *The Exerciser's Handbook.* New York: David McKay Co., Inc., 1978.

Kushner, Rose. "Breast Self-Examination (BSE): Tips and Guides." *Breast Cancer—National Women's Health Network Resource Guide I*, Washington, D.C., 1981.

Labrum, Anthony H. "Depression and Feminine Endocrine Pathology." Unpublished paper, University of Rochester School of Medicine and Dentistry, Department of Obstetrics-Gynecology and Psychiatry, 1984.

Lane, J. M., Vigorita, V. J., and Falls, M. "Osteoporosis, Current Diagnosis and Treatment." *Geriatrics*, vol. 39, no. 4, Apr. 1984:40–47.

Lanson, Lucienne, T. "Urinary Disorders." *Better Homes and Gardens Woman's Health and Medical Guide.* Des Moines, Iowa: Meredith Corp., 1981:148–160.

——. "Adult Reproductive Problems." *Better Homes and Gardens Woman's Health and Medical Guide.* Des Moines, Iowa: Meredith Corp., 1981:471–484.

La Rocca, Susan A. and Polit, Denise, F. "Women's Knowledge About the Menopause." *Nursing Research*, vol. 29, no. 1, Jan.–Feb. 1980:10–13.

Laufer, Larry R., Erlik, Yohanan, Meldrum, David R., and Judd, Howard L. "Effect of Clonidine on Hot Flashes in Postmenopausal Women." *Obstetrics and Gynecology*, vol. 60, no. 5, Nov. 1982:583–586.

Lecos, Chris. "A Compendium on Fats." *FDA Consumer.* Reprinted from Mar. 1983, HHS Publication No. (FDA) 83-2171.

Leiblum, Sandra, Bachmann, Gloria et al. "Vaginal Atrophy in the Post-menopausal Woman: The Importance of Sexual Activity and Hormones." *Journal of the American Medical Association*, vol. 249, no. 16, Apr. 22/29, 1983:2195–98.

Lennon, Mary Clare. "The Psychological Consequences of Menopause: The Importance of Timing of a Life Stage Event." *Journal of Health and Social Behavior*, vol. 23, no. 4, Dec. 1982:353–366.

Lettvin, Maggie. *Maggie's Woman's Book.* Boston: Houghton, Mifflin Co., 1980.

Levinson, Ilene S. "Research Briefs." *Midlife Wellness*, vol. 1, no. 3, 1983:44–46.

——. "Research Briefs." *Midlife Wellness*, vol. 1, no. 4, 1984:55/57–58.

Lewis, Vaughn. "Getting the Most of the F Complex." *Prevention*, vol. 36, no. 9, Sept. 1984:48–54.

Lloyd, Charles W. "Sexuality in the Climacteric." *The Menopause: Comprehensive Management.* Edited by Bernard A. Eskin. Masson Publishing, Inc., 1980:101–110.

Logan, Wende. "Questions I Always Wanted to Ask—But Didn't." *Midlife Wellness*, vol. 2, no. 2, 1985:85–87.

Lopez, Maria Cristina, Costlow, Judy, Adams, Edith, Romero, Pita, Gladfelter, Jeanne, and Morrison, Maggie. *Menopause: A Self-Care Manual.* Santa Fe, New Mexico: Santa Fe Health Education Project, 1980.

Love, Susan M., Gelman, Rebecca Sue, and Silen, William. "Fibrocystic 'Disease' of the Breast—A Non-Disease?" *New England Journal of Medicine,* vol. 307, no. 16, Oct. 14, 1982:1010–1014.

Luce, Gay G. and Peper, Erik. "Learning How to Relax." *Stress.* Chicago: Blue Cross Association 1984:84–94.

Machol, Libby. "Postmenopausal Osteoporosis: New Approaches to Prevention." *Contemporary Ob/Gyn,* vol. 20, Aug. 1982:153–161.

MacPherson, Kathleen. "Hot Flash: The Menopause Collective." *Sojourner,* Feb. 1981:11.

———. "Menopause As Disease: The Social Construction of a Metaphor." *ANS/Women's Health,* 1981:95–113.

Madaras, Lynda and Patterson, Jane. *Womancare.* New York: Avon Books, 1981.

Maddox, Hilary C. *Menstruation.* New Canaan, Conn.: Tobey Publishing Company, 1975.

Marks, R. and Shahrad, P. "Aging and the Effect of Estrogens on the Skin." *The Menopause: A Guide to Current Research and Practice.* Baltimore: University Park Press, 1976:144–161.

Martin, Leonide. *Health Care of Women.* Philadelphia: J. B. Lippincott Co., 1978.

Masters, William H. and Johnson, Virginia E. *Human Sexual Inadequacy.* Boston: Little Brown & Co., 1980.

———. *Human Sexual Response.* Boston: Little Brown & Co., 1966.

Maxmen, Jerold S. *A Good Night's Sleep.* New York: W. W. Norton & Co., 1981.

McCalls. "When Breast Lumps Aren't Cancer," May 1985:65–66.

McGoldrick, Kathryn E. "Myths, Menopause and Middle Age," editorial. *Journal of the American Medical Woman's Association,* vol. 37, no. 4, 1982:86.

McKenzie, Lynda. "Osteoporosis Related Hip Fractures: The Financial Cost." *Midlife Wellness,* vol. 1, no. 4, 1984:68–69.

McKinlay, Sonja, Jeffreys, Margot, and Thompson, Barbara. "An Investigation of the Age At Menopause." *Journal of Biological Science,* vol. 4, 1972:161–173.

McQuade, Walter and Aikman, Ann. *Stress.* New York: E. P. Dutton & Co., Inc., 1974.

Medical World News. "Workshop Findings Inconclusive on Estrogen, CHD Link," Nov. 14, 1983:22–23.

Meldrum, David R. "Perimenopausal Menstrual Problems." *Clinical Obstetrics and Gynecology,* vol. 26, no. 3, Sept. 1983: pp. 762–768.

Menopause Update. "Research Briefs: Continuous Treatment with Hormones for Climacteric Complaints." vol. 1, no. 1, Fall 1982:36.

———. "Vaginal Estrogen Cream Usage and its Absorption." vol. 1, no. 2, 1983: 47.

——. "Premature Bone Loss in Non-Menstruating Women" and "Thyroid Supplements May Decrease Bone Mass." vol. 1, no. 1, Fall 1982:35.

——. "High Calcium Intake Associated with Decrease in Blood Pressure." "Zinc Deficiency May Result From Long-Term Use of Diuretics." "Premenstrual Tension Occurs in Climacteric Women." "Vaginal Estrogen Cream Usage and Its Absorption." vol. 1, no. 2, 1983:45–47.

——. "Salt: How Much is Too Much?" vol. 1, no. 1, Fall 1982: 28–32.

——. "News Briefs: American Cancer Society Recommendations for Breast Cancer Screening." vol. 1, no. 1, Fall 1982:38.

Midlife Wellness. "Research Briefs: Biopsy and Aspiration." vol. 2 no. 2, 1985:107–109.

——. "Hormone Pellet Implants: A Pictorial Description." vol. 1, no. 3, 1983:18–20.

——. "Do Estrogens Control Rapid Bone Loss?" and "Lower Extremity Loading and Bone Formation." vol. 2, no. 1, 1983" 46–47.

Miller, M. A., Drakontides, A. B., and Leavell, L. C. *Kimber-Gray-Stackpole's Anatomy and Physiology*, 17th Edition. New York: Macmillan Publishing Co., 1977.

Miller, Roger W. "On Being Too Rich, Too Thin, Too Cholesterol Laden." *FDA Consumer.* Reprinted from July/Aug. 1981, HHS Publication no. (FDA) 81–1087.

Millette, Brenda and Hawkins, Joellen. *The Passage Through Menopause.* Reston, Va.: Reston Publishing Co., Inc., 1983.

Mirkin, Gabe. "Unwelcome Hair." *Health*, July 1982.

Molnar, George W. "Body Temperatures During Menopausal Hot Flashes." *Journal of Applied Physiology*, vol. 38, no. 3, Mar. 1975:499–503.

Morell, Martha J., Dixen, Jean M., Carter, C. Sue, and Davidson, Julian M. "The Influence of Age and Cycling Status on Sexual Arousability in Women." *American Journal of Obstetrics and Gynecology*, vol. 148, no. 1, Jan. 1, 1984:66–71.

Morgan, Susanne. *Coping With a Hysterectomy.* New York: The Dial Press, 1982.

Nachtigall, Lila E. "Hormone Therapy: Benefits Versus Risks." *Midlife Wellness*, vol. 1, no. 3, 1983:29–37.

Napoli, Maryann. "Breast Cancer: The Truth About Early Detection." *Ms.*, May 1983:86–89.

——. "Breast Cancer: An Update." *Network News*, vol. 8, no. 4, July/Aug., 1983:2–7.

National Cancer Institute. *Breast Cancer: We're Making Progress Every Day*, NIH Publication No. 83-2409, 1983.

——. *Breast Exams: What You Should Know.* NIH Publication No. 82-2000, 1981.

National Dairy Council. "Diet, Nutrition and Cancer." *Dairy Council Digest*, vol. 54, no. 6, Nov./Dec., 1983:31–36.

——. "The Role of Calcium In Health." *Dairy Council Digest*, vol. 55, no. 1, 1984:1–8.

——. "Weight Control." *Dairy Council Digest*, vol. 55, no. 2, Mar./Apr., 1984:9–14.

National Dairy Council Publications. *The All-American Guide to Calcium-Rich Foods*, 1984.

——. *For Mature Eaters Only*, 1984.

——. *Guide to Wise Food Choices*, 1982.

——. *To Your Health . . . In Your Second Fifty Years*, 1983.

——. *What to Know About a Weight-Control Diet Before You Eat One*, 1981.

——. *Are You at Risk for Bone Disease?*, 1984.

——. *Calcium—You Never Outgrow Your Need for It*, 1984.

——. *Like Mother, Like Daughter: A Woman's Guide to Bone Health*, 1985.

——. *Sticks and Stones Can Break Your Bones . . . And So Will Too Little Calcium*, 1985.

National Institute on Aging. "Age Page/Osteoporosis: The Bone Thinner." Dec. 1983.

——. "Aging and Your Eyes." Sept. 1983.

——. "Skin—Getting the Wrinkles Out of Aging." Mar. 1981.

——. "Age Page: Taking Care of Your Teeth," Sept. 1981.

——. "Osteoporosis and Aging." Prepared for the 1981 White House Conference on Aging.

National Institutes of Health. *The Menopause Time of Life*, brochure, NIH Publication No. 83-2461, Sept. 1983.

——. U.S. Department of Health and Human Services. "Osteoporosis, Cause, Treatment, Prevention," April 1983.

National Society for the Prevention of Blindness, Inc., publications. *The Aging Eye*, July, 1974.

——. *Glaucoma*, Feb. 1977.

——. *Your Eyes . . . for a Lifetime of Sight*, Sept. 1976.

Natow, Annette and Heslin, Jo-Ann. *Nutrition for the Prime of Your Life.* New York: McGraw-Hill, 1983.

Neugarten, Bernice L. and Kraines, Ruth J. "'Menopausal Symptoms' in Women of Various Ages." *Psychosomatic Medicine*, vol. 27, no. 3, 1965:266–273.

Neugarten, Bernice L., Wood, Vivian, Kraines, Ruth J., and Loomis, Barbara. "Women's Attitudes Toward the Menopause." *Vita Humana*, vol. 6, 1963:140–151.

Newsweek. "Keeping Fit for Life," Aug. 6, 1984:63–64.

——. "New Comforts for Old Bones," Sept. 17, 1984:79.

——. "Cancer: A Radical Departure," Mar. 25, 1985:91.

The New York Times. "Estrogens May Make Heart Disease More Likely," Mar. 20, 1984:2.

Nolan, William A. "Estrogen Therapy At Menopause: Weighing the Risks." *McCall's*, May 1981:59–60.

Nordon, B. E. Christopher. "Bone Loss at the Menopause." *Menopause Update*, vol. 1, no. 1, Fall, 1982:5–9.

Norris, Ronald V. and Sullivan, Colleen. *PMS: Premenstrual Syndrome.* New York: Rawson Associates, 1983.

Notelovitz, Morris. "Estrogen, Lipids and Coronary Heart Disease—A Hypothesis." *Midlife Wellness*, vol. 1, no. 3, 1983:38–41.

———. "Menopause: When to Treat." *Menopause Update*, vol. 1, no. 2, 1983:27–31.

Notelovitz, Morris and Ware, Marsha. *Stand Tall! The Informed Woman's Guide to Preventing Osteoporosis.* Gainesville, Fla.: Triad Publishing Co., 1982.

Notelovitz, Morris, Whitehead, M. I., Gambrell, R. Don, Jr., and Dinnerstein, Lorraine. "Forum Highlights: Menopause, Role of Hormone Therapy (Part I: Hormone Replacement)." *The Female Patient*, vol. 8, July 1983:50/28–40/41.

Ob. Gyn. News. "Fluoride Held Theory of Choice in Postmenopausal Osteoporosis," Jan. 1–14, 1984:12–13.

Offit, Avodah. "Sexuality: The Facts of (Later) Life." *Ms.*, Jan., 1982:32.

Pak, Charles, Y. C. "Postmenopausal Osteoporosis." *The Menopause.* Edited by Herbert J. Buchsbaum. New York: Springer-Verlag, 1983:35–54.

Pariza, Michael W. "A Perspective on Diet, Nutrition and Cancer." *Journal of the American Medical Association*, vol. 251, no. 11, Mar. 16, 1984:455–458.

Parsons, C. Lowell and Schmidt, Joseph D. "Control of Recurrent Lower Urinary Tract Infection in the Postmenopausal Woman." *The Journal of Urology*, vol. 128, no. 6, Dec. 1982:1224–1226.

Pearson, Linda. "Climacteric." *American Journal of Nursing*, vol. 82, no. 7, July 1982:1098–1102.

Pedersen, Bonnie and Pendleton, Elaine. "Menopause: A Welcome or Dreaded Stage of Development." *Journal of Nurse Midwifery*, vol. 23, Fall 1978:45–51.

People. "Osteoporosis, The 'Silent' Disease, Strikes One in Four Women Over 65, An Expert Warns," April 1, 1985:129.

Perlmutter, Ellen and Bart, Pauline B. "Changing Views of 'The Change': A Critical Review and Suggestions for an Attributional Approach." *Changing Perspectives in Menopause.* Edited by A. M. Voda, M. Dinnerstein, and S. R. O'Donnell. Austin: University of Texas Press, 1982:187–197.

Petitti, Diana B. "Menopausal Estrogens and Vascular Diseases." *Midlife Wellness*, vol. 1, no. 3, 1983:9–12.

Phillips, Elliott Richard. *Get a Good Night's Sleep.* Englewood Cliffs, N.J.: Prentice-Hall, Inc., 1983.

Physician's Desk Reference 1984. Oradell, N.J.: Medical Economics Co., Inc., 1984.

Pinkham, Mary Ellen. "The Best Exercise of All . . . Which You Are Probably Already Doing." *Ms.*, May 1983:59.

Planned Parenthood of Rochester and Monroe County. "Menopause." Brochure distributed 1984.

——. *My Menopause: Program Guide.* Rochester, N.Y.: Education Department Publications.

Planned Parenthood of Syracuse, Inc. *Feeling Fit in the Forties and Fifties,* 1980.

Porcino, Jane. *Growing Older, Getting Better.* New York: Addison-Wesley Publishing Co., 1983.

Ravnikar, Veronica A., Schiff, Isaac, and Regestein, Quentin R. "Estrogen Improves Sleep Via Abatement of Vasomotor Symptoms." *The Menopause.* Edited by Herbert J. Buchsbaum. New York: Springer Verlag, 1983:161–171.

Redbook. "The Supersmoothers," June 1984:18.

Regestein, Quentin R. with Rechs, James R. *Sound Sleep.* New York: Simon & Schuster, 1980.

Reimer, Lisa. "Nutrition and Cancer—A Brief Overview." *Midlife Wellness,* vol. 1, no. 4, 1984:13–19.

Reitz, Rosetta. *Menopause: A Positive Approach.* Radnor, Pa.: Chilton Book Co., 1977.

Rhinehart, John S. and Schiff, Isaac. "Hormone Imbalance: Hormone Treatment?" *Menopause Update,* vol. 1, no. 2, 1983:13–16.

Richelson, Linda S., Wahner, Heinz W., Melton, L. J. III, and Riggs, B., Lawrence. "Relative Contributions of Aging and Estrogen Deficiency to Postmenopausal Bone Loss." *The New England Journal of Medicine,* vol. 311, no. 20, Nov. 15, 1984:1273–75.

Roen, Leah J. "Environmental Variables Influencing Osteoporosis." *Midlife Wellness,* vol. 1, no. 3, 1983:51–55.

Rose, Louisa, ed. *The Menopause Book.* New York: Hawthorn Books, 1977.

Rosenfeld, Anne Harris. "Aging." *Better Homes and Gardens Woman's Health and Medical Guide.* Des Moines, Iowa: Meredith Corporation, 1981:324–329.

Sarrel, Philip M. and Lorna J. "Sexuality in the Middle Years." *Menopause Update,* vol. 1, no. 1, Fall 1982:25–29.

Schiff, Isaac. "The Effects of Progestins on Vasometer Flushes." *The Journal of Reproductive Medicine,* vol. 27, no. 8, Aug. 1982:498–502.

——, Regestein, Quentin, Tulchinsky, Dan, and Ryan, Kenneth J. "Effect of Estrogens on Sleep and Psychological State of Hypogonadal Women." *Journal of the American Medical Association,* vol. 242, no. 22, Nov. 30, 1979:2405–07.

Science News. "Estrogen for Curbing Bone Loss?," vol. 125, no. 5, Apr. 14, 1984:238.

Seaman, Barbara and Seaman, Gideon. *Women and the Crisis in Sex Hormones.* New York: Bantam Books, 1977.

Seidman, Herbert, Stellman, Steven D., and Moshinski, Margaret H. "A Different Perspective on Breast Cancer Risk Factors: Some Implications of the Non-Attributable Risk." *Journal for Clinicians*, vol. 2, no. 5, 1982. (reprint distributed by the American Cancer Society)

Seltzer, Vicki Lynn. "Sex and Medical Care After Menopause." *American College of Obstetricians and Gynecologists* Newsletter, May 10, 1983.

Semmens, James P. "Sexuality." *The Menopause*. Edited by Herbert J. Buchsbaum. New York: Springer-Verlag, 1983:175–180.

Semmens, James P. and Wagner, Gorm. "Estrogen Deprivation and Vaginal Function in Postmenopausal Women." *Journal of the American Medical Association*, vol. 248, no. 4, July 23/30, 1982:445–448.

Severne, Liesbeth. "Psychosocial Aspects of the Menopause." *Changing Perspectives on Menopause*. Edited by Ann M. Voda, Myra Dinnerstein, and Sheryl R. O'Donnell. Austin: University of Texas Press, 1982:239–247.

Shainess, Natalie. "Menopause: Midlife Crisis or Milestone Marker?" *Journal of the American Medical Women's Association*, vol. 37, no. 4, April 1982:87–90.

Shangold, Mona M. "Sports and Exercise." *The Menopause*. Edited by Herbert J. Buchsbaum. New York: Springer-Verlag, 1983:199–203.

Sheehy, Gail. *Pathfinders*. New York: William Morrow and Co., Inc., 1981.

——. *Passages*. New York: E. P. Dutton & Co., Inc., 1976.

Shephard, Bruce. "Do You Really Need a Hysterectomy?" *McCall's*, Aug. 1974:140–142.

Shephard, Bruce D. and Shephard, Carroll A. *The Complete Guide to Women's Health*. Tampa, Fla.: Mariner Publishing Co., 1982.

Shimizu, Holly, H. "Do Yourself A Flavor." *FDA Consumer*. Reprinted from April, 1984, HHS Publication No. (FDA) 84-2192.

Silberner, J. "Breast Cancer: Death to the Radical?" *Science News*, vol. 127, no. 11, Mar. 16, 1985:165.

Sillence, David. "Osteoporosis and the Osteoporosis of Osteogenesis Imperfecta." Presentation at the First National Conference of the American Brittle Bone Society, a report distributed in 1984.

Sitruk-Ware, Regine. "Newer and Alternative Methods of Hormone Administration." *Midlife Wellness*, vol. 1, no. 3, 1983:13–17.

Soules, Michael R. and Bremner, William J. "The Menopause and Climacteric: Endocrinologic Basis and Associated Symptomology." *Journal of the American Geriatrics Society*, vol. 30, no. 9, Sept. 1982:547–561.

Spellacy, William N. "Abnormal Bleeding." *Clinical Obstetrics and Gynecology*, vol. 26, no. 3, Sept. 1983:702–707.

Stare, Fredrick J. and Whelan, Elizabeth M. "Nutrition." *Better Homes and Gardens Woman's Health and Medical Guide*. Des Moines, Iowa: Meredith Corporation, 1981:40–59.

Starr, Bernard D. and Weiner, Marcella B. *The Starr-Weiner Report on Sex and Sexuality in the Mature Years*. New York: Stein and Day, 1981.

State of New York, Department of Health. *Estrogen/The Risks and Benefits*, brochure, Nov. 1981.

Stein, Gerald H. "Breast Self Examination: A New Training Method." *Midlife Wellness*, vol. 2, no. 2, 1985:91–94.

Steinem, Gloria. "Fifty Is What 40 Used to Be—and Other Thoughts on Growing Up." *Ms.*, vol. 12, no. 12, June 1984:108–110.

Stevenson, Dallas and Delprato, Dennis J. "Multiple Component Self-Control Program for Menopausal Hot Flashes." *Journal of Behavior Therapy and Experimental Psychiatry*, vol. 14, no. 2, June, 1983:137–140.

Stewart, Felicia, Guest, Felicia, Stewart, Gary, and Hatcher, Robert. *My Body My Health*. New York: John Wiley and Sons, 1979.

Stumpf, Paul G. "The Estradiol Vaginal Ring." *Midlife Wellness*, vol. 1, no. 3, 1983:21–23.

Swenson, Norma. "Breast Cancer: The Problem." *Breast Cancer—Resource Guide I*. Washington, D.C.: National Women's Health Network, 1981.

Thompson, Irene. "The Widow in American Society." *Midlife Wellness*, vol. 1, no. 3, 1983:24–28.

Time. "Is Male Menopause A Myth?," vol. 114, no. 8, Aug. 20, 1979:68.

Tucker, Sherry Jill. "The Menopause: How Much Soma and How Much Psyche?" *JOGN Nursing*, Sept./Oct. 1977:40–48.

Upton, Virginia G. "Therapeutic Considerations in the Management of the Climacteric: A Critical Analysis of Prevalent Treatments." *The Journal of Reproductive Medicine*, vol. 29, no. 2, Feb. 1984:71–79.

Utian, Wulf H. "Current Status of Menopause and Postmenopausal Estrogen Therapy." *Obstetrical and Gynecological Survey*, vol. 32, no. 4, 1977:193–204.

——. *Menopause in Modern Perspective*. New York: Appleton-Century-Crofts, 1980.

——. "Vaginal Function in Postmenopausal Women." Letter in *Journal of the American Medical Association*, vol. 249, no. 2, Jan. 14, 1983:194–195.

U.S. Department of Agriculture, U.S. Department of Health and Human Services. "Sodium, Think About It." *Home and Garden Bulletin*, no. 237, May 1982.

U.S. Department of Health, Education and Welfare. "To Be or Not to Be An Estrogen User? Summary of Conclusions of the NIH Consensus Development Conference on Estrogen Use and Postmenopausal Women," Sept. 13–14, Bethesda, Maryland, 1979.

U.S. Department of Health and Human Services. "Some Facts and Myths of Vitamins." *FDA Consumer*. Reprinted from Sept. 1979, HHS Publication No. (FDA) 79-2117.

U.S. Department of Health and Human Services, National Institutes of Health. *Cancer Prevention*. NIH Publication No. 84-2671, Feb. 1984.

Voda, Ann M. "Hot Flushes/Flashes, A Descriptive Analysis." *Menopause Update*, vol. 1, no. 2, 1983:17–20.

——. "Menopausal Hot Flash." *Changing Perspectives on Menopause*. Edited by A. M. Voda, M. Dinnerstein, and S. R. O'Donnell. Austin: University of Texas Press, 1982:136–159.

Voet, Richard L. "End Organ Response to Estrogen Deprivation." *The Menopause.* Edited by Herbert J. Buchsbaum. New York: Springer-Verlag, 1983:9–22.

Ware, Marsha. "Does Vitamin E Help Hot Flashes?" *Menopause Update,* vol. 1, no. 1, Fall 1982:33.

——. "Breast Changes After Menopause Makes Mammograms Easier to Interpret." *Midlife Wellness,* vol. 2, no. 2, 1985:114.

——. "Osteoporosis—The Brittle Bone Disease." Savvy, April 1983:104–108.

——. "Research Briefs: Patient-Physician Cooperation Key to Early Breast Cancer." *Midlife Wellness,* vol. 2, no. 2, 1984:113.

Washington State Dairy Council. *Osteoporosis,* 1984.

Weideger, Paula. *Menstruation and Menopause.* New York: Alfred A. Knopf, 1976.

Weinshelbaum, Arlene and Weinshelbaum, Edward. "Mammography." *Midlife Wellness,* vol. 2, no. 2, 1985:98–102.

Whitehead, Malcolm I. "Long-Term Usage of Hormones . . . Is it Beneficial in Preventing Postmenopausal Osteoporosis?" *Midlife Wellness,* vol. 1, no. 3, 1983:2–8.

Whitfield, William. "Breaking the Habit." *Nursing Mirror,* September 8, 1982:59–60.

Williams, Charlotte. "A Woman's Perspective . . . Menopause." *Menopause Update,* vol. 1, no. 1, Fall, 1983:15–19.

Wilkin, Jonathan K. "Flushing Reactions: Consequences and Mechanisms." *Annals of Internal Medicine,* vol. 95, no. 4, 1981:468–476.

Willis, Judith. "Diet Books Sell Well But . . ." *FDA Consumer.* Reprinted from Mar. 1982, HHS Publication No. (FDA) 82-1093.

Willet, W., Stampfer, M. J., Bain, C. et al. "Cigarette Smoking, Relative Weight and Menopause." *American Journal of Epidemiology,* vol. 117, no. 6, 1983:651–656.

Wilson, Robert A. *Feminine Forever.* New York: M. Evans and Co., Inc., 1966.

Women's Health Network. "Old Problem, New 'Disease.' The Controversy Surrounding Pre-Menstrual Syndrome." *Network News,* Summer 1984:5–6.

Woods, Nancy Fugate. "Menopausal Distress: A Model for Epidemiologic Investigation." *Changing Perspectives on Menopause.* Edited by A. M. Voda, M. Dinnerstein, and S. R. O'Donnell. Austin: University of Texas Press, 1982:220–238.

The World Almanac and Book of Facts 1984. Cites data from National Center for Health Statistics, U.S. Dept. of Health and Human Services, New York, Newspaper Enterprise Association, Inc.

World Health Organization. "Research on the Menopause." *The Lancet,* vol. 2, no. 8290, July 17, 1982:137–138.

Xerox Corporation. *Take Charge Health Management Program Fitbook,* 1980.

Zauner, Christian, W. "Exercise: A Health Care Need." *Midlife Wellness,* vol. 1, no. 4, 1984:33–43.

Zussman, Leon, Zussman, Shirley, Sunley, Robert, and Bjornson, Edith. "Sexual Response After Hyst-oophorectomy: Recent Studies and Reconsideration of Psychogenesis." *American Journal of Obstetrics and Gynecology,* vol. 140, no. 7, Aug. 1, 1981:725–729.

Index

About the Author

Susan Flamholtz Trien was born in Brooklyn, New York, and graduated cum laude from Brooklyn College in 1969. She is currently a full-time writer and lives in Rochester, New York, with her husband and their two children.

Formerly with Maternity Center Association in New York City, Ms. Trien developed educational materials for expectant parents and was associate editor of the agency's medical news magazine. She has written extensively on women's health issues for national magazines, and is also author of *Parents Book of Breastfeeding*.